SPEECH SYNTHESIS AND RECOGNITION

J.N. Holmes
Speech Technology Consultant
Formerly Head of the Joint Speech Research Unit

 Van Nostrand Reinhold (UK) Co. Ltd

First published in 1988 by
Van Nostrand Reinhold (UK) Co. Ltd.
Molly Millars Lane, Wokingham, Berkshire, England

Typeset in 10/12 pt Times by
Witwell Ltd, Liverpool

Printed and bound in Great Britain by
T.J. Press (Padstow) Ltd, Padstow, Cornwall

British Library Cataloguing in Publication Data
Holmes, J. N.
   Speech synthesis and recognition. —
   (Aspects of information technology).
   1. Automatic speech recognition   2. Speech
   synthesis
   I. Title   II. Series
   006.4′54   TK7882.S65

   ISBN 0-278-00013-4

CONTENTS

PREFACE

As information technology continues to make more impact on many aspects of our daily lives, the problems of communication between human beings and information-processing machines become increasingly important. Up to now such communication has been almost entirely by means of keyboards and screens, but there are substantial disadvantages in this method for many applications. Speech, which is by far the most widely used and natural means of communication between people, is at first sight an obvious substitute. However, this deceptively simple means of exchanging information is, in fact, extremely complicated. Although the application of speech in the man–machine interface is growing rapidly, in their present forms machine capabilities for generating and interpreting speech are still a travesty of what a young child can achieve with ease. This volume sets out to explain why the problem is so difficult, how it is currently being tackled, and what is likely to happen in the future as our knowledge and technological capability improve. It does not attempt to cover the human factors aspects of using speech for the man–machine interface, as this is another specialism.

This book is intended as an introduction to and summary of the current technology of speech synthesis and recognition. It is most appropriate as a text for those graduate students or specialist undergraduates in information technology who have an electronic engineering or computer science background. Although the book should be useful for people trained in other disciplines, such as linguistics or psychology, some additional reading on signal processing mathematics and electronic technology would probably be necessary for such readers to derive the maximum benefit.

This volume should also be suitable as background material for electronic engineers in industry who need to apply their skills to engineering speech technology products, and for systems engineers who wish to use speech technology devices in complete information processing systems.

An advanced mathematical ability is not required, although it is assumed the reader has some familiarity with the basic mathematics of electronic engineering, such as Fourier analysis, convolution, continuous and discrete-time filters, etc. No specialist knowledge of phonetics or of the properties of speech signals is assumed. Chapter 8, which describes the application of hidden Markov models to speech recognition, requires some statistics knowledge – in particular elementary probability theory and the properties of the normal distribution. I believe that for those trying to understand hidden Markov models for the first time, a large part of the problem arises from the difficulty of remembering the meanings of the symbols used in the equations. For this reason the symbols adopted in Chapter 8 are different from those used almost universally in research papers in this field. Instead they have been made to have some mnemonic association with the quantities they describe. Once the form of the equations has become familiar and their significance is understood, the reader should have no difficulty in transferring to the standard notation, using a, b, α and β.

Although this book explains some of the basic concepts in great detail, a volume of this size cannot hope to give a comprehensive coverage of speech synthesis and recognition. It should, however, provide sufficient information to enable the reader to understand many of the current research papers in this area. The subjects described owe a lot to numerous published papers by many different authors over the last 50 years. Study of these papers should not be necessary for the reader to follow the explanations given here, and to simplify the text only a few important original sources of some of the subjects have been referenced directly. However, in Chapter 11 there is a bibliography containing sufficient information to enable readers with more specialist interests to trace all the significant literature in any of the fields covered.

For much of my knowledge in the subjects covered in this book, I am greatly indebted to all of my many colleagues and other associates in the field of speech research, particularly during the long period I was in the Joint Speech Research Unit. In preparing the book I have received much useful advice and detailed help from Andy Downton, in his role as a series editor. I also wish to express by special gratitude to Norman Green, Wendy Holmes, Martin Russell and Nigel Sedgwick, who made valuable constructive comments on drafts of various chapters.

1

HUMAN SPEECH COMMUNICATION

1.1 VALUE OF SPEECH FOR MAN–MACHINE COMMUNICATION

Developments in electronic and computer technology are causing an explosive growth in the use of machines for processing information. In most cases this information originates from a human being, and is ultimately to be used by a human being. There is thus a need for effective ways of transferring information between people and machines, in both directions. One very convenient way for this communication in many cases is in the form of speech, because speech is the communication method most widely used between humans; it therefore seems extremely natural and requires no special training.

There are, of course, many circumstances where speech is not the best method for communicating with machines. For example, large amounts of text are much more easily received by reading from a screen, and positional control of features in a computer-aided design system is easier by direct manual manipulation. However, for interactive dialogue and for input of large amounts of text or numeric data speech offers great advantages. For all applications where the machine is only accessible from a standard telephone instrument there is no practicable alternative.

1.2 IDEAS AND LANGUAGE

To appreciate how communication with machines can use speech effectively, it is important to understand the basic facts of how humans use speech to communicate with each other. The normal aim of human speech is to communicate ideas, and the words and sentences we use are not usually important as such. However, development of intellectual activity and language acquisition in human beings proceed in parallel in early childhood, and the ability of language to code ideas in a convenient form for mental processing and retrieval means that to a large extent people actually formulate the ideas themselves in words and sentences. The use of language in this way is only a convenient coding for the ideas. Obviously a speaker of a different language would code the same concepts in different words, and different individuals within one language group might have quite different shades of meaning they normally associate with the same word.

1.3   THE RELATIONSHIP BETWEEN WRITTEN AND SPOKEN LANGUAGE

Invention of written forms of language came long after humans had established systems of speech communication, and individuals normally learn to speak long before they learn to read and write. However, the great dependence on written language in modern civilization has produced a tendency for people to consider language primarily in its written form, and to regard speech as merely a spoken form of written text – possibly inferior because it is imprecise and often full of errors. In fact, spoken and written language are different in many ways, and speech has the ability to capture subtle shades of meaning that are quite difficult to express in text, where one's only options are in choice of words and punctuation. Both speech and text have their own characteristics as methods of transferring ideas, and it would be wrong to regard either as just an inferior substitute for the other.

1.4   PHONETICS AND PHONOLOGY

The study of how human speech sounds are produced and how they are used in language is an established scientific discipline, with a well developed theoretical background. The field is split into two branches: the actual generation and classification of speech sounds falls within the subject of **phonetics**, whereas their function in languages is the concern of **phonology**. These two subjects need not be studied in any detail by students of speech technology, but there are phonetic and phonological aspects of the generation and use of speech that must be appreciated in general terms. The most important ones are covered briefly in this chapter and in Chapter 2.

1.5   THE ACOUSTIC SIGNAL

The normal aim of a talker is to transfer ideas, as expressed in a particular language, but putting that language in the form of speech involves an extremely complicated extra coding process (Fig. 1.1). The actual signal

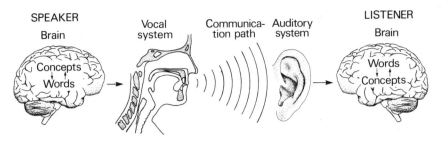

Fig. 1.1 Illustration of the processes involved in communicating ideas by speech. It is not easy to separate the concepts in the brain from their representation in the form of language.

transmitted is predominantly acoustic, i.e. a variation of sound pressure with time. Although particular speech sounds tend to have fairly characteristic properties (better specified in spectral rather than waveform terms), there is great variability in the relationship between the acoustic signal and the linguistic units it represents. In analysing an utterance linguistically the units are generally discrete, e.g. words, phrases, sentences. In speech the acoustic signal is continuous, and it is not possible to determine a precise mapping between time intervals in a speech signal and the words they represent. Words normally join together, and in many cases there is no clear acoustic indication of where one word ends and the next one starts. For example, in the sequence 'six seals' the final sound of the 'six' is not significantly different from the [s] at the beginning of 'seals', so the choice of word boundary position will be arbitrary. All other things being equal, however, one can be fairly certain that the [s] sound in the middle of 'sick seals' will be shorter, and this duration difference will probably be the only reliable distinguishing feature in the acoustic signal for resolving any possible confusion between such pairs of words. The acoustic difference between 'sick seals' and 'six eels' is likely to be even more subtle.

Although the individual sound components in speech are not un-ambiguously related to the identities of the words, there is, of course, a high degree of systematic relationship that applies most of the time. Because speech is generated by the human vocal organs (explained further in Chapter 2) the acoustic properties can be related to the positions of the articulators. With sufficient training, phoneticians can, based entirely on listening, describe speech in terms of a sequence of events related to articulatory gestures. This auditory analysis is largely independent of age or sex of the speaker. The International Phonetic Alphabet (IPA) is a system of notation whereby phoneticians can describe their analysis as a sequence of discrete units. Although there will be a fair degree of unanimity between phoneticians about the transcription of a particular utterance, it has to be accepted that the parameters of speech articulation are continuously variable, so there will obviously be cases where different people will judge a particular stretch of sound to be on the opposite sides of a phonetic category boundary.

1.6 PHONEMES, PHONES AND ALLOPHONES

Many of the distinctions that can be made in a narrow phonetic transcription, for example between different people pronouncing the same word in slightly different ways, will have no effect on meaning. For dealing with the power of speech sounds to make distinctions of meaning it has been found useful in phonology to define the **phoneme**, which is the smallest unit in speech where substitution of one unit for another might make a distinction of meaning. For example, in English the words 'do' and 'to' differ in the initial phoneme, and 'dole' and 'doll' differ in the middle (i.e. the vowel sound). There may be many different features of the sound pattern that contribute to the phonemic distinction: in the latter example, although the tongue position during the vowel would normally be slightly different, the most salient feature in choosing between the two words would probably be vowel duration. A similar inventory of symbols is used for phonemic notation as for the more detailed phonetic transcription, although the set of phonemes is specific to the language being described. For any one language only a small subset of the IPA symbols is used to represent the phonemes, and each symbol will normally encompass a fair range of phonetic variation. There are about 44 phonemes in English, the precise number and the choice of symbols depending on the type of English being described (i.e. some types of English fail to make phonetic distinctions between pairs of words that are clearly distinct in others). It is usual to write phoneme symbols between oblique lines, e.g. /t/, but to use square brackets round the symbols representing the sound of a particular manifestation of a phoneme (known as a **phone**).

Many of the IPA symbols are, in fact, the same as characters of the Roman alphabet, and frequently their phonetic significance is similar to that commonly associated with the same letters in those languages that use this alphabet. To avoid the need to give details of the IPA notation in this book, the use of IPA symbols will in general be restricted to characters whose phonemic significance should be obvious to speakers of English.

There is a wide variation in the acoustic properties of phones representing a particular phoneme. In some cases these differences are merely the result of the influence of neighbouring sounds on the positions of the tongue and other articulators. This effect is known as **co-articulation**. In other cases the difference might be a feature that has developed for the language over a period of time, which new users learn as they acquire the language in childhood. An example of the latter phenomenon is the vowel difference in the words 'coat' and 'coal' as spoken in southern England. These vowels are acoustically quite distinct, and use a slightly different tongue position. However, they are regarded as **allophones** of the same phoneme because they are never used as alternatives to distinguish between words that would otherwise be identical. Substituting one vowel for the other in either word would not cause the word identity to change, although it would certainly give a pronunciation that would sound odd to a native speaker.

1.7 VOWELS AND CONSONANTS

We are all familiar with the names **vowel** and **consonant** as applied to letters of the alphabet. Although there is not a very close correspondence in English between the letters in conventional spelling and their phonetic significance, the categories of vowel and consonant are, for the most part, similarly distinct in spoken language.

During vowels the flow of air through the mouth and throat is relatively unconstricted, whereas in most consonants there is a substantial constriction to air flow for some of the time. In some consonants, known as **stop consonants** or **plosives**, the air flow is completely blocked for a few tens of milliseconds. Although speech sounds that are classified as vowels can usually be distinguished from consonants by this criterion, there are some cases where this distinction is not very clear. It is probably more useful to distinguish between vowels and consonants phonologically, on the basis of how they are used in making up the words of a language. Languages show a tendency for vowels and consonants to alternate, and sequences of more than three or four vowels or consonants are comparatively rare. By considering their functions and distributions in the structure of language it is usually fairly easy to decide, for each phoneme, whether it should be classified as a vowel or a consonant. There are some cases where the different phonological structure will cause phonetically similar sounds to be classified as vowels in one language and consonants in another.

1.8 PHONEMES AND SPELLING

It is very important in the study of speech not to be confused by the conventional spelling of words, particularly for English where the relationship between spelling and pronunciation is so unpredictable.

Although the vowel/consonant distinction in English orthography is not very different from that made in phonetics and phonology, there are obvious anomalies. In the word 'gypsy', for example, the two examples of the letter y are both functioning as vowels, whereas in 'yet' the y is clearly a consonant.

The letter x in the word 'vex' represents a sequence of two consonants (it would be transcribed phonemically as /**veks**/), but gh in 'cough' represents a single phoneme, /**f**/.

There are many cases in English where the letter e after a consonant is not pronounced, but its presence modifies the phonemic identity of the vowel before the consonant (such as 'dot' and 'dote'). Combinations of vowel letters are often used to represent a single vowel phoneme (such as in 'bean') and in several varieties of English a letter r after a vowel is not pronounced as a consonant but causes the vowel letter to represent a different phoneme ('had' changes to 'hard' and 'cod' to 'cord').

In English there are many vowel phonemes that are formed by making a transition from one vowel quality to another, even though they function as single phonemes in the phonological system. Such vowels are known as **diphthongs**. The vowel sounds in 'by', 'boy' and 'bough' are typical examples, and no significance should be assigned to the fact that one is represented by a single letter and the others by 'oy' and 'ough'.

1.9 PROSODIC FEATURES

The identities of the phonemes are not the only carriers of linguisic information in speech. An important role in human speech communication is also played by pitch, intensity and timing. In some languages, of which Chinese is the most obvious example, the pattern of pitch variation within a word is needed to supplement knowledge of the phonemes to determine the word's identity. In Chinese there are four different **tones** which can be used, representing four patterns of pitch change. In most European languages pitch, duration and intensity (collectively known as the **prosodic** features of the speech) do not normally affect the identities of the words, but they do provide important additional information about what is being said.

Prosodic features can be used to indicate the mood of the speaker, and to emphasize certain words. Prosody is also the main factor responsible for determining which syllables are stressed in polysyllabic words. The most salient prosodic feature for indicating stress and word prominence is not, as one might expect, intensity but is in fact pitch – in particular the change of pitch on stressed syllables. Sound duration also increases for stressed syllables, but there are many other factors that affect durations of sounds, such as their positions in a sentence and the identities of the neighbouring sounds. Although prominent syllables do tend to be slightly more intense, and low-pitched sounds at the ends of phrases are often a few decibels weaker, intensity is less significant in assisting speech interpretation than are pitch and duration.

By focusing attention on the most important words, correct prosody is a great help in the interpretation of spoken English. Speech in which the prosody is appreciably different from that normally used by a native speaker can be extremely difficult to understand. Although the detailed variations of pitch pattern vary considerably between different local English accents (for example, between London and Liverpool), the general way in which prosody is used to mark stress is similar. With some other languages, however, such as French, the rhythmic structure is completely different. In such **syllable-timed** languages the syllables seem to come in a much more uniform stream than in **stress-timed** languages such as English, where there often seems to be a regular 'beat' on the main stressed syllables. The implication is that in English the unstressed syllables between the syllables carrying the most prominence are shorter if there are more of them. Although this difference of type of rhythm between English and French is clearly perceived by listeners, there has been much controversy over its physical correlates. Attempts to find a systematic difference between the measured patterns of syllable durations of English and French in spontaneous conversation have not been very successful.

1.10 LANGUAGE, ACCENT AND DIALECT

Different languages often use quite different phonetic contrasts to make phonemic distinctions. This fact causes great difficulty for foreign language learners, particularly if their speech habits are already firmly established in their native language before another is encountered. It is beyond the scope of this book to give details of this effect, but a simple example will illustrate the point. In Japanese there is no phoneme corresponding to the English $/l/$, but there is one that is acoustically somewhere between English $/l/$ and $/r/$, normally regarded as a type of $/r/$. When most Japanese hear an [l] in English it does not sound very close to any sound in their own language, but it is perceptually nearer to the sound associated with their $/r/$ than to any other. Speech is used for transmitting language, and there is a strong tendency to sub-consciously replace one's memory of a speech sound by its linguistic label (i.e. phoneme) within a second or two of hearing it uttered. It is very common, therefore, for Japanese to be unable to distinguish, in both perception and production, between English words that differ only by an $/l/ - /r/$ contrast (e.g. 'light' and 'right'). This comment is not to be interpreted as a criticism specifically of foreign speakers of English, because native English speakers have similar difficulties, particularly in distinguishing vowel contrasts in languages with a very rich vowel system such as Swedish.

Different **accents** of the same language, although they may have just as much acoustic difference as different languages between representations of the equivalent phonemes, do not normally cause much difficulty for native speakers. Because the underlying linguistic structure is almost identical, there are not many cases where the differences of phonetic quality between accents actually cause confusion in the intended word. For example, Scottish English would not distinguish between the vowels in 'good' and 'food', but this does not cause confusion to southern English listeners because in this case the intended word (in their own accent) will be nearest perceptually to what they hear. Even when there is a possible word confusion (such as in the identical southern English pronunciations of 'flaw' and 'floor', which would be clearly distinct in Scottish), there is usually enough context available for only one of the word candidates to make sense.

The term **dialect** is often used to indicate clearly different varieties, spoken by a substantial group of people, of what is basically the same language. In addition to having appreciable variations of pronunciation, as in the examples above, dialects are often also associated with the use of alternative words and sometimes grammatical changes, which are not encountered outside the area where the dialect is spoken.

1.11 SUPPLEMENTING THE ACOUSTIC SIGNAL

It is apparent from the comments above that when humans listen to speech they do not hear an unambiguous sequence of sounds, which can be decoded one by one into phonemes and grouped into words. In many cases, even for an unambiguous sequence of phonemes, there is ambiguity about the sequence of words. (Consider the sentences: 'It was a grey day.' and 'It was a grade A.') In fluent speech it will frequently be the case that the sound pattern associated with phonemes, particularly in unstressed positions, will not be sufficiently distinct from the sound of alternative phonemes for the intended word to be clear. In normal conversation false starts to words, hesitation, and mild stuttering are extremely common. In the presence of background noise or a reverberant environment the speech signal might be further distorted so that distinctions that were clear at the speaker's mouth are no longer so at the listener's ear. Yet people do, in fact, manage to communicate by speech extremely easily.

In normal language there is so much redundancy in the linguistic message that only a small fraction of the information potentially available is necessary for the listener to deduce the speaker's meaning (even if, in some cases, there will be uncertainty about some of the minor words). All sorts of information is taken into account by the listener. This information will include what the listener knows about the speaker, and therefore what he/she is likely to talk about. If the conversation has already been in progress for some time, there will be a very strong influence from the previous context. Once the listener has got used to the speaker's voice, allowance will be made for his/her particular accent in resolving some phonemic ambiguities. But most of all, for each sentence or phrase, the listener will choose the one interpretation that seems to make most sense taking all available information into account, both acoustic and contextual. In some cases the decision will actually involve rejecting some phonemes which accord well with the acoustic signal, in favour of others which would seem less likely based on the acoustic evidence alone. Except when the acoustic evidence is very much at variance with the norm for the chosen phoneme, the listener will not usually even be aware that the acoustic pattern was not quite right. By analogy, when people read printed text minor typographical errors are frequently unnoticed, and the intended words are perceived as though they were really there.

Most people are familiar with the fact that in a crowded room, such as at a cocktail party, they can converse with the group of people in their immediate vicinity, even though there is a lot of competing speech at a high acoustic level from all the other people in the room. There is extra information in this case that is not available, for example, when listening through a telephone receiver. In the first place the availability of two ears enables some directional discrimination to be used. The human hearing system has an ability to infer direction by using the difference in intensity and time of arrival at the two ears of sounds which have otherwise similar structure.

The other important factor in face-to-face communication is the ability to see the speaker, and to correlate the acoustic signal with observed lip movements, and with other gestures which may be used to supplement the speech. Although it is usual to associate lip reading with deaf people, those with normal hearing generally develop a high degree of sub-conscious ability to integrate visual information with auditory signals to assist them in decoding speech. This lip-reading ability will not often be sufficient on its own to resolve what has been said, but it is of great value in selecting between consonant sounds that may be easily confusable in background noise using only the acoustic signal, yet have very distinct lip movements.

To the newcomer to this subject, the most surprising thing is perhaps that the listener is completely unaware of this integration of visual with auditory information. The subjective impression to the listener is of actually 'hearing' the acoustically ambiguous stimulus correctly, and the joke about partially deaf people putting on their glasses so that they can hear better is a reality. In fact this same phenomenon of integration of knowledge sources to contribute to one's perception of the words 'heard' applies to all knowledge, including linguistic knowledge and knowledge of the influence of the real world on what people are likely to say.

1.12   THE COMPLEXITY OF SPEECH PROCESSING

It is clear that the human perceptual and cognitive systems must be enormously complex to be able to perform the task of linguistic processing. The very large number of neurons are, of course, working in parallel, so the fact that the actual processing speed in any one part of the central nervous system is very slow compared with the speed of modern electronic cirucits does not prevent the overall perceptual decisions from being made within a few hundreds of milliseconds. Where machines are required to recognize and interpret speech, it is apparent that emulating human performance in processing normal relaxed conversation will not be possible without the machine having a very high degree of artificial intelligence and extensive linguistic knowledge. However, if the task of the machine is simplified by placing constraints on the speech that is spoken, it is already possible to use speech for many types of man–machine interaction. Developments currently in progress will greatly increase the range of tasks for which speech is useful.

Even so, the situation so often depicted in science fiction, where machines seem to have no difficulty at all in understanding anything that people say to them, is still many years away.

SUMMARY
Chapter 1

The use of speech offers great advantages for many types of man-machine communication, particularly by telephone. Understanding how humans use speech highlights some of the problems.

Speech is mainly used to communicate ideas, and the ideas are normally formulated in the brain in the form of language. Spoken and written language are quite different in their capabilities.

Phonetics is the study of the production and properties of speech sounds, and phonology is the study of how they are used in language. The relationship between the acoustic properties of a speech signal and the linguistic units it represents is extremely complicated, and often leaves ambiguity in interpretation which can only be resolved by using other information.

The individual speech sounds (phones) are physical realizations of the smallest linguistic units (phonemes) of a speech signal. Allophones are different sounds that represent the same phoneme; the choice of allophone usually depends on local phonetic context.

In speech, vowels and consonants can be defined according to their phonetic properties, but it is more useful to take into account their phonological functions also. The classification of vowels and consonants, and determination of the sequence of phonemes, is often only slightly related to conventional spelling of a language, particularly for English.

Pitch, intensity and timing collectively make up the prosodic features of speech, which supplement the phonetic properties. Prosody is valuable for indicating important words, and adding emotional content to a message. Pitch change is the most salient prosodic feature, and intensity variations are less important than timing.

Phonetic features are used differently in different languages, and people cannot usually detect phonetic differences which are not used in their native language. Various accents of the same language also show phonetic variation, but with the same underlying linguistic structure these variations do not usually cause serious problems in comprehension.

In human speech comprehension all available information is used to supplement the phonetic properties of the speech. This information includes the direction of the sound source, lip movements and other gestures where these can be seen, and extensive knowledge of the language, context, and the state of the world, all of which influence what words are likely to be heard next.

The human speech perception and production processes are so complicated that their full capabilities will not be emulated mechanically for many years. However, for many more limited speech generation and recognition applications there are already extremely useful machines, and their capabilities are rapidly being improved.

EXERCISES
Chapter 1

E1.1 Give examples of circumstances where speech would not be the best medium for man-machine communication, and other circumstances where there is a great advantage in using speech, or perhaps no practical alternative.

E1.2 What is the difference between phonetics and phonology?

E1.3 Explain, with examples, why it is often not possible to unambiguously divide a speech signal into separate words unless the identities of the words are already known.

E1.4 Explain the relationship between phonemes, phones and allophones.

E1.5 What factors contribute to the distinction between vowels and consonants?

E1.6 Discuss the role of prosody in speech communication.

E1.7 Why is speech communication often possible even when the speech signal is extremely distorted?

2

MECHANISMS AND MODELS OF HUMAN SPEECH PRODUCTION

2.1 INTRODUCTION

When developing speech synthesis and recognition systems for their many possible applications, the task is made much easier if one has a good understanding of how humans generate speech, and how the various human processes can be modelled by electric circuits or in a computer. A speech generation model, in addition to aiding understanding of speech production, can in itself form the basis of a speech synthesis system.

The main organs of the human body responsible for producing speech are the **lungs, larynx, pharynx, nose** and various parts of the **mouth**, which are illustrated by the cross-section shown in Fig. 2.1. Muscular force to expel air from the lungs provides the source of energy. The air flow is modulated in various ways to produce components of acoustic power in the audio frequency range. The properties of the resultant sound are modified by the rest of the vocal organs to produce speech.

The process of acoustic resonance is of prime importance in determining the properties of speech sounds. The principal resonant structure, particularly for vowels, is know as the **vocal tract**; it starts at the larynx and extends up through the pharynx and mouth to the lips. For some sounds the nose is also coupled in to make a more complicated resonant system. The frequencies of the resonances and the way they move with time, and to a lesser extent their intensities, are crucial in determining what is being said. The main resonant modes of the vocal tract are known as **formants**, and by convention they are numbered from the low-frequency end. For conciseness they are usually

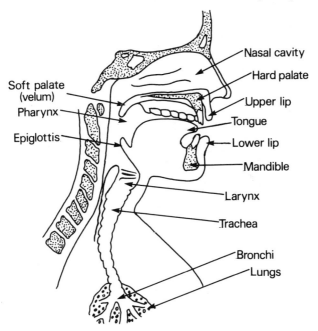

Fig. 2.1 Diagrammatic cross-section of the human head, showing the vocal organs.

referred to as F_1, F_2, F_3, etc. In general F_1 and F_2 (normally in the range 250 Hz to 3 kHz) are the most significant in determining the phonetic properties of speech sounds, but some higher-frequency formants can also be important for some phonemes.

2.2 SOUND SOURCES

The air stream from the lungs can produce three different types of sound source to excite the acoustic resonant system. These various sound sources are brought into operation according to what type of speech sound is being produced.

For **voiced** sounds, which normally include all vowels and some consonants, such as [m, n, l, w,], the air flow from the lungs and up the trachea is modulated by vibrations of the **vocal folds**, located in the larynx. The vocal folds (sometimes also known as the vocal cords) are illustrated in Fig. 2.2. They are two folds of tissue stretched across the opening in the larynx. The front ends of the folds are joined to the thyroid cartilage, and the rear ends to the arytenoid cartilages. The arytenoids can, under muscular control, move far apart so that there is a wide triangular opening between the vocal folds. This is the normal condition for breathing. They can also bring the folds tightly

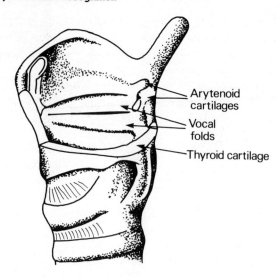

Fig. 2.2 Cut-away view of the human larynx.

together, completely closing the top of the trachea. This condition is achieved when one holds one's breath, and it occurs automatically during swallowing, to prevent food or drink from entering the lungs. The arytenoids can also be held so that the vocal folds are almost touching. If air is forced through the slit-like opening between them (known as the **glottis**), the folds will start to vibrate, and so modulate the air flow. There will then be a build-up of vocal fold oscillation whose frequency is mainly determined by the mass and tension of the folds, but is also affected by the air pressure from the lungs. The modulation of the air stream by the vibrating vocal folds is known as **phonation**. When the vibration amplitude has built up sufficiently, which usually happens after one or two cycles, there is enough movement for the vocal folds to make contact in the closing phase, thus completely and abruptly stopping the air flow.

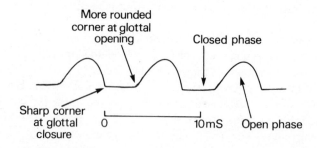

Fig. 2.3 Typical air-flow waveform through the glottis during phonation.

The variation of volume flow through the glottis is typically as shown in Fig. 2.3. The presence of a sharp corner at the point of closure gives rise to a power spectrum of the air-flow waveform with frequency components of significant (though small) magnitude up to several kilohertz. It is thus the shock to the resonant system resulting from the sudden blocking of the air flow through the glottis that causes the main excitation of the formants in every phonation cycle. The fundamental frequency of this signal lies typically in the range 50–200 Hz for adult male speakers, and about one octave higher for adult females. The subjective impression of voice pitch is very closely related to the fundamental frequency, and is only slightly affected by the formant frequencies. Although the spectrum of a single glottal pulse will have a continuous distribution in frequency, the periodic repetition of pulses will cause the total voiced excitation to approximate to a line spectrum.

Besides the gradual build-up of phonation described above, it is also possible for phonation to start with the vocal folds held just in contact. In this case the build-up of pressure starts the process by forcing the folds apart to allow the first glottal pulse through, but within two or three cycles the vibration will settle into a periodic pattern, similar to that which occurs when the folds are slightly apart at the start of phonation. With a closed-glottis start, the formants will even be excited by the closure of the first glottal pulse.

The cessation of phonation can also have two distinct patterns, depending on whether the folds are relaxed and pulled apart, or are forced tightly together. In the former case the vibration dies out gradually, with the folds not touching in the last few cycles. In the latter, the pulses cease very quickly but the glottal closure remains sharp, even in the last pulse. In addition, the last two or three pulses before cessation are usually further apart in time. Firmly closing the glottis to stop phonation for a few tens of milliseconds, and then allowing phonation to re-start suddenly by relaxing the closing force, produces the so-called **glottal stops** that are a characteristic feature of many people's speech in, for example, London and Glasgow.

The overall complexity of the vocal fold vibration differs for different people, and the shape of the flow waveform varies with vocal effort and other aspects of voice quality. For example, sometimes the parting of the vocal folds is sufficiently fast for there to be significant power in the higher audio frequencies at that part of the cycle also. In addition to the actual air flow through the glottis, there are other small components of the effective volume velocity into the bottom of the pharynx that arise from surface movements of the vocal folds. During phonation the whole of the vocal fold structure moves up and down as well as laterally. On glottal closure there is a rippling motion of the upper vocal fold surface which causes additional air displacement just above the larynx during the closed period. The volume displacement caused by this effect is small compared with the total volume of a glottal pulse, and its influence on the low-frequency power (i.e. the lowest two or three harmonics) is negligible. However, these surface movements are fairly rapid (involving times of the order of 1 ms). At higher frequencies, where the energy associated with the sharpness of glottal closure is only a very small fraction of the total pulse energy, this additional source of volume flow can significantly modify the spectral components of glottal excitation. In some circumstances it might contribute to the characteristic voice qualities of different speakers, although such effects will be small compared with other speaker-specific factors affecting voice quality.

The second major source of sound in speech production is the air turbulence that is caused when air from the lungs is forced through a constriction in the vocal tract. Such constrictions can be formed in the region of the larynx, as in the case of [h] sounds, and at many other places in the tract, such as between various parts of the tongue and the roof of the mouth, between the teeth and lips, or between the lips. The air turbulence source has a broad continuous spectrum, and the spectrum of the radiated sound is affected by the acoustics of the vocal tract, as in the case of voiced sounds. Sustainable consonant sounds that are excited primarily by air turbulence, such as [s, f], are known as **fricatives**, and in consequence the turbulence noise is often referred to as **frication**.

The third type of sound source results from the build-up of pressure that occurs when the vocal tract is closed at some point for a stop consonant. The subsequent plosive release of this pressure produces a transient excitation of the vocal tract which causes a sudden onset of sound. If the vocal folds are not vibrating during the closure, the onset is preceded by silence. If the vocal folds are vibrating during the pressure build-up the plosive release is preceded by low-level sound; the power of this sound is mostly at the fundamental frequency of phonation, and is radiated through the walls of the vocal tract. The plosive release approximates a step function of pressure, with its consequent –6 dB/octave spectrum shape, but its effect is of very short duration and the resultant excitation merges with the turbulent noise at the point of constriction, which normally follows the release.

In connected speech all of these sound sources are brought into play as a result of muscular control, with just the right timing for them to combine, in association with the appropriate dimensions of the resonant system, to produce the complex sequence of sounds that we recognize as a linguistic message. For many sounds (such as [v, z]) the voiced excitation from the vocal folds occurs simultaneously with turbulent excitation. It is also possible to have turbulence generated in the larynx during vowels to achieve a breathy voice quality. This quality is produced by not closing the arytenoids quite so much as in normal phonation, and by generating the vibration with a greater air flow from the lungs. There will then be sufficient random noise from air turbulence in the glottis combined with the periodic modulation of the air flow to produce a characteristic breathiness that is common for some speakers. If this effect is taken to extremes, a slightly larger glottal opening, tense vocal folds and more flow will not produce any phonation, but there will then be enough turbulence at the larynx to produce whispered speech.

2.3   THE RESONANT SYSTEM

In the discussion that follows, the concepts of acoustic resonance, coupling, damping, impedance, etc. are widely used. For electrical engineers these concepts in acoustics are not normally familiar, but they are, in fact, very closely analogous to their electrical counterparts, and it can therefore be helpful to think of them in electrical terms. In acoustic systems it is normal to regard sound pressure as analogous to voltage, and volume flow as analogous to current. Energy loss as a result of viscosity is then represented by series electrical resistance, and heat conduction losses can be associated with shunt conductance. The inertance of a mass of air corresponds to inductance, and compliance of the air to capacitance.

Using these concepts the theory of sound transmission in the vocal tract is very similar to electrical transmission line theory, and the major structural discontinuity at the larynx end can be fairly well modelled by appropriate lumped values of resistive and reactive components.

If the **soft palate** (or **velum**) is raised and held in contact with the rear wall of the pharynx there will be no opening between the pharynx and nose; the properties of the vocal tract between larynx and lips can then be modelled fairly closely by an unbranched air-filled tube with a large number of cylindrical sections butted together. Assuming the cross dimensions of this tube are such that there is only plane wave propagation along its length at audio frequencies, and assuming sound propagation within the tube is entirely without loss, it is not too difficult to calculate the response of such a tube, i.e. the mathematical transfer function relating volume velocity inserted at the larynx end to that radiated from the lips. The mathematics becomes

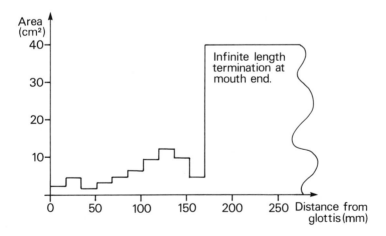

Fig. 2.4   Graph of cross-section of a 10-section acoustic tube modelling a typical vowel. The mouth termination is shown coupling into an infinite tube of cross-section 40 cm^2.

more practical if, instead of radiating into free space, the lip opening is represented as coupling into an infinite-length tube of cross-section that is large compared with the opening, as illustrated in Fig. 2.4. The detailed analysis of this situation is beyond the scope of this book, but it is given by Rabiner and Schafer (1978), pp. 92–98.

The results of this analysis show that the transfer function is periodic in frequency, with a repetition every $cN/2L$, where c is the velocity of sound, N is the number of elementary tubes and L is the total length of the model tract. As any transfer function for a real system must have a frequency response that is symmetrical about zero frequency, the periodicity implies there is also symmetry about odd multiplies of $cN/4L$. A typical response is shown in Fig. 2.5. The frequency-domain periodicity is exactly the same as occurs in sampled-data filters, and is evident in the s-plane to z-plane transformation that is used in sampled-data filter theory. The relevance of sampled-data filter theory is a consequence of the fact that a wave travelling in an abutted set of uniform tubes only has any disturbance to its propagation when it meets a change in diameter, to cause partial reflection. As these changes occur at regular distances, and therefore at regular time intervals, the response must be representable by a sampled-data system, which has a sampling rate of $cN/2L$ (i.e. the sampling interval is equal to twice the wave propagation time through one tube section). The reason for the factor of 2 is that the minimum time before any partial reflection can again influence the conditions at any tube junction is equal to the time taken for the reflected component to return to the previous junction, and then be reflected back to the point under consideration.

For a sound velocity of 350 m/s, and a tract length of 0.175 m (typical for an adult male speaker) a total of 10 elementary tubes will specify a total of 5 resonances within the range 0 – 5 kHz, which will be the 5 lowest formants of the system. There will, however, be mirrored and repeated resonances at higher frequencies, which will be very unlikely to fit the real speech spectrum above 5 kHz. A greater number of tube sections would enable the resonant

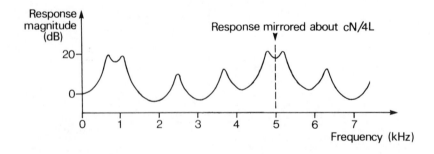

Fig. 2.5   Typical response of a 10-section acoustic tube, such as is illustrated in Fig. 2.4.

modes to be independently specified up to a higher frequency, and could be represented by a sampled-data filter with a higher sampling rate.

The transfer function of the acoustic tube model has an infinite number of poles, but no zeros. The magnitude of the transfer function is directly related to the frequencies of the poles, and when the dimensions of the tube are such that two resonant modes move close in frequency, the intensities associated with these resonances will increase. If the tube is uniform the resonances will be equally spaced, at $c/4L, 3c/4L, 5c/4L$, etc., and the magnitude of the transfer function will be the same at each resonant frequency.

There are many idealizing assumptions associated with the above calculations, many of which do not fit the facts of human speech production very closely. However, this acoustic tube model will predict the frequencies of the three or four lowest formants in the vocal tract fairly well if the cross-sectional area is known as a function of distance along the tract. The model will not describe the high frequencies at all well, for a number of reasons. First, the assumption of plane waves is only valid when the cross dimensions of the tubes are small compared with a half-wavelength of sound. This assumption will be seriously in error at some places in the tract from about 3 kHz upwards. Second, the complexities of shape around, for example, the epiglottis, the sides of the tongue, the teeth, etc., are totally unlike the abutted cylindrical tubes of the model. Third, there are significant losses in the vocal tract from many causes. These losses will give rise to an increase of damping of the resonances, and in particular the higher frequency resonances will become very heavily damped because the reflection from the mouth opening will not be so effective for wavelengths comparable with the mouth dimensions.

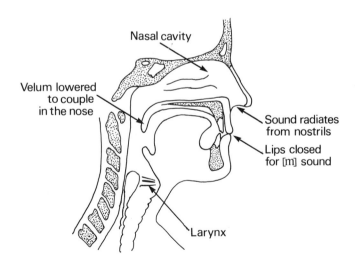

Fig. 2.6   Acoustic system for producing a typical nasal consonant, [m].

For nasal consonants, e.g. [m, n], the soft palate is lowered to produce appreciable coupling between the top of the pharynx and the nose. In addition, the mouth is blocked at some point determined by the identity of the consonant. There will thus be a branched acoustic system, illustrated in Fig. 2.6, with a closed side branch (the mouth). Apart from the effect of vocal tract wall vibrations, all the sound will come out of the nose. Mathematical analysis then becomes much more difficult, partly because of the unknown and variable coupling at the velar opening, but even more because of the very complicated structure of the nasal cavities. Apart from the division into two parts by the nasal septum, the inside of the nasal cavities has elaborately shaped bony structures, some acoustic coupling into the sinus cavities, and a considerable quantity of hair around the nostrils. The effect of all of these features is to increase the damping of the resonances, to increase the total number of resonant modes in a given frequency range, and to cause spectral zeros as well as poles in the transfer function as a result of the side branch.

It is also possible to have the velum lowered during vowel sounds, to produce **nasalized vowels**. In languages such as French the nasalized vowels are distinct phonemes, and the change to the properties of the acoustic signal as a result of nasalization is very noticeable. In other languages, such as English, nasality in vowels has no linguistic significance. However, because specific muscular effort is required to keep the velum raised to decouple the nose, it is common for there to be a considerable degree of nasal coupling during English vowels, particularly adjacent to nasal consonants. The most prominent acoustic effect is to cause an additional resonance near to the first formant, and to cause additional first formant damping. Nasalization in

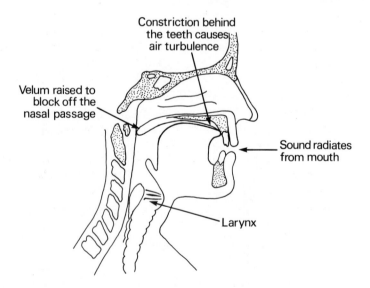

Fig. 2.7   Articulator positions for producing the fricative consonant, [s].

vowels is not so common near to fricative or plosive consonants, because the velum has to be raised to allow the pressure build-up needed during consonant production.

The resonant frequencies (and therefore the poles of the transfer function) of the vocal tract for a given configuration are independent of the position of the sound source. However, there are three differences which make the spectral envelope of the radiated sound very different for voiced excitation, compared with plosive or fricative excitation. First, the spectrum of the voiced source has nearly all of its power in the lowest few harmonics, and the slope of the spectral intensity above about 1 kHz is at least − 12 dB/octave. At low vocal effort the fall-off is often a lot faster. Second, the vocal tract is much less constricted for most of the time during voiced sounds, except at the glottis, where it is closed or almost closed. During voiceless sounds the glottis is normally fairly wide open, such that the acoustic system behind the source of frication includes the sub-glottal system. Because of the coupling with the bronchi and the lungs, this system is quite heavily damped. The third effect is that (except when the constriction is in the laryngeal region) the sound source is further forward in the vocal fract. Fig. 2.7 illustrates a typical vocal tract configuration for producing the sound [s].

There are two alternative ways of analysing the effect of the different position of the sound source. One way is to consider the whole acoustic system, which has transfer function poles that are independent of the placement of the source. That part of the vocal tract behind the source acts as though it were a closed tube in series with the source to the total system, and its transfer function poles will cause absorption of power from the source at the pole frequencies, and thus add zeros at these frequencies to the transfer function from source to lips. However, as there is normally a close constriction at any point of frication or stop release, the acoustic systems on each side of the constriction are almost independent (i.e. there is very little coupling between them). In these cirumstances the poles of the overall system are almost the same as the poles of the two part-systems considered in isolation; the poles associated with the part of the tract behind the constriction will thus be almost coincident with the zeros, and will therefore have their effects substantially cancelled. It is then possible to regard the tract length as consisting only of the part from the constriction to the lips, and to ignore the part behind the constriction. This shorter vocal tract will, of course, have more widely spaced resonances, and for sounds where the constriction is very near the mouth opening (e.g. [s, f]) the resonant length will be so short and the ratio of mouth opening to cavity volume will be so large that there will be only one or two obvious resonant modes, tuned to high frequencies (above 3.5 kHz) and very broad because of their heavy damping.

2.4 INTERACTION BETWEEN THE LARYNGEAL AND VOCAL TRACT FUNCTIONS

During voiceless sounds, where the glottis is normally wide open, there is strong acoustic coupling between the vocal tract and the sub-glottal system. However, as explained above, the constriction needed to produce excitation for these sounds substantially decouples the region behind the constriction, and so the sub-glottal system has very little effect on the acoustics of the radiated sound. In the case of sounds excited primarily by the glottal air flow, the time-varying impedance presented by the glottis to the lower end of the pharynx will affect the overall sound properties. Of course, the transfer function relating volume flow at the glottis to sound radiated from the lips does not depend on glottal opening, but the finite acoustic impedance at the glottis when it is open will mean that the volume flow through the glottis will depend on the frequency-dependent load impedance presented by the vocal tract. In consequence there can be prominent ripple components of the open-phase glottal flow at the formant frequencies, particularly for F_1. It is easier to appreciate the effects of the varying glottal impedance, not by taking into account this modification to the effective source waveform, but by estimating the effect of the glottal impedance on the poles of the whole acoustic system, which includes the glottis. An electrical equivalent circuit of the acoustic system is shown in Fig. 2.8.

The impedance looking down the trachea below the glottis will be fairly low, because of the large cross-sectional area and the heavy damping on any resonances caused by the structure of the lungs. Even at its maximum opening in the phonatory cycle the glottis area is very much smaller than that of the trachea, so the acoustic impedance presented to the bottom of the pharynx is substantially that of the glottis itself. The impedance will be a combination of resistance, and reactance resulting from the mass of the air in the glottal opening. The effect of the open-glottis impedance for typical vowels is to cause a small increase of F_1 frequency, but a very noticeable increase of F_1

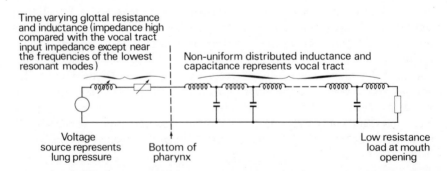

Fig. 2.8 Electrical equivalent circuit of the glottis coupled to an idealized vocal tract, with all losses at the terminations.

damping. The higher formants, which are more heavily damped anyway because of other losses, show much smaller effects.

When looking at the speech waveform for the period from one main glottal excitation point to the next, it is not at all easy to know whether to attribute observed departures from a simple decaying resonant system response to variations in glottal impedance, or to changes in volume flow stemming directly from phonation. For example, if the vocal folds part sharply enough at the beginning of their open phase, the start of the glottal flow can cause significant secondary excitation of F_1, which may be in such a phase relationship to the decaying F_1 response from the previous glottal closure that it causes partial cancellation, producing a sudden reduction in amplitude. It would be difficult in such a case to distinguish the effect from that caused by a sudden increase of formant damping. The same phenomenon occurring with slightly different phonation or formant frequencies might cause an amplitude increase which would be clearly seen as secondary excitation, and would normally be followed by an obvious increase in rate of amplitude decay because of the extra damping. The extra formant damping in the open-glottis period is most noticeable for open vowels, such as the [ɑ] sound in the first syllable of 'father'. These vowels have a smaller pharynx cross-section, which is more closely matched to the glottal area, so substantially reducing wave reflections at the glottis. When the glottis is closed, the damping of F_1 is such that the 3-dB bandwidth of the formant is about 50 Hz, but for the open glottis it can be at least four times greater. Typical closed-glottis bandwidths for F_2 are around 80 Hz, and for the higher formants can be 150 Hz or more.

In addition to glottal opening having an effect on F_1, F_1 can also have some effect on the glottis. If a low-order harmonic of the fundamental frequency of phonation is near the frequency of F_1, the F_1 flow through the glottis causes a slight tendency for the relaxation oscillation of the vocal folds to be 'pulled' by the formant frequency, thus making the harmonic move with the formant.

Another interaction between the fundamental frequency and the formants occurs because the muscular force needed to raise the pitch also raises the larynx. (This movement might be as much as 20 mm.) The raising of the larynx shortens the pharynx, and thus tends to increase the formant frequencies. This modification to the formant frequencies is one reason why it is possible to perceive pitch changes even when speech is whispered.

2.5 RADIATION

So far the discussion has been on the properties of the sound sources, and the effect of the resonant system on the properties of the volume velocity at the lips and nostrils. The volume flow leaving these openings causes a pressure wave to be radiated, which can be heard by a listener or cause a response from a microphone. The waveform shape of the radiated pressure wave from a small opening in a large baffle can be found by taking the time derivative of

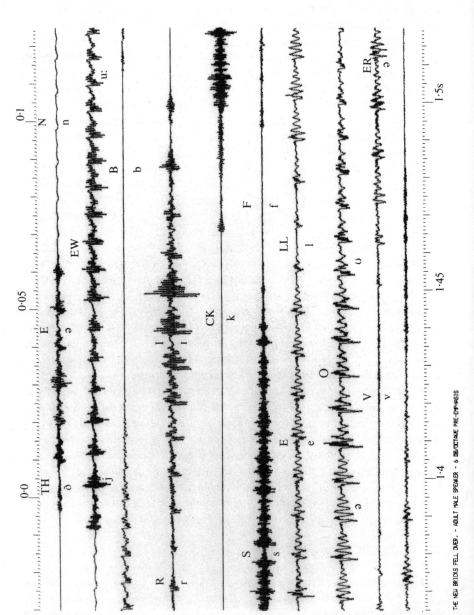

Fig. 2.9 Waveform of the sentence 'The new bricks fell over' spoken by an adult male southern British talker. Although the sentence is only 1.5 s long the time scale is too compressed to show the detail. The text is marked above the graph in conventional orthography, and below in phonemic notation, both in approximate time alignment with the waveform.

the volume flow from the radiating orifice. The spectrum of the radiated sound therefore differs from that of the volume velocity by a 6 dB/octave lift. When the mouth and nose are both radiating at the same time (in nasalized vowels) the two pressure waves will combine. At all frequencies where the audio power is significant the wavelength will be so great compared with the spacing between mouth and nostrils that simple addition of the volume velocities from the two sources will suffice. Diffraction round the head will reduce the level in front of the head by up to 3 dB for wavelengths large compared with the head dimensions, because a significant fraction of the power at these frequencies will be radiated behind the speaker. However, this level change is fairly small compared with the effect of the wide variety of different acoustic environments that the human listener is easily able to allow for. For example, the low-frequency spectrum drop can be largely compensated by having the speaker stand with his/her back to a wall, and a low-frequency boost would be caused when a speaker stands facing outwards from a corner.

2.6 WAVEFORMS AND SPECTROGRAMS

An annotated typical speech waveform, representing the sentence 'The new bricks fell over' spoken by an adult male with a southern British accent, is shown in Fig. 2.9. The variety of structure associated with the various speech sounds is very obvious, and some information about the phonetic content can be derived from waveform plots. However, the waveform is not useful for illustrating the properties of speech that are most important to the general sound quality or to perception of phonetic detail. In view of the importance in speech communication of resonances and their time variations, some means of displaying these features is needed. The short-time spectrum of the signal, equivalent to the magnitude of a Fourier transform of the waveform after it has been multiplied by a time-window function of appropriate duration, cannot of course, show any information that is not in the original signal. It will, however, be more suitable for displaying the resonances. Because the time variations of the resonances are responsible for carrying the phonetic information that results from moving the articulators, it is important that a means be available for displaying a succession of Fourier transforms at short time intervals (e.g. at most a few milliseconds apart).

There are many ways in which a succession of Fourier transforms can be displayed. Using current computer technology, the speech waveform for analysis could be input to the computer using an analogue-to-digital converter, and the required Fourier transforms could be calculated and plotted, each one just below the next, on a screen or on paper. This method of spectral analysis can be useful for some purposes, but it is not easy to interpret formant movements from such a succession of spectral cross-sections, partly because when they are plotted far enough apart to be distinguishable, the total amount of display area needed for even a fairly short sequence of phonetic events is excessive. It has been found much easier for general study of the acoustic properties of speech signals to use the horizontal dimension for time, the vertical dimension for frequency, and to represent the short-time spectral intensity at each frequency by visual intensity, or colour, or some combination of the two. In this way it is possible to get a very compact display of a few seconds of speech in a way in which the phonetically important acoustic features can easily be interpreted. It is obviously not possible to judge relative intensities of different parts of the signal so precisely from such a variable intensity display as it would be from a spectral cross-section plot, but in practice a variable intensity plot is usually adequate for most purposes. If a combined colour and intensity scale is available it is, of course, possible to get finer spectral level discrimination.

So far the discussion has assumed that a computer and Fourier transforms will be used for generating **spectrograms**. This method is computationally very expensive, but is is widely used in research laboratories with very good computing facilities. The earliest spectrograms (in the 1940s) were, however, made by purpose-built **spectrographs** to obtain equivalent pictures by a completely different technique. The magnitude of the short-time Fourier transform at a particular frequency and time is exactly equivalent to the signal amplitude at the appropriate time from a suitable band-pass filter centred on the required frequency. The width and shape of the filter pass-band have to be chosen so that the envelope of its impulse response corresponds to the time window used on the input to the Fourier transform.

The original spectrographs stored a few seconds of speech on a magnetic drum so that it could be played back repetitively. On the same shaft as the magnetic drum was another drum, on which was wrapped a sheet of electro-sensitive paper. Held in contact with the paper was a stylus mounted on a slide driven by a screw geared to the drum. When a sufficient voltage was applied to the stylus, the resultant sparking caused the paper to burn, so turning it black. For each revolution of the drum the stylus moved along by about 0.25 mm, so that it eventually covered the whole surface of the paper. The movement of the stylus was also used to vary the frequency of a heterodyne oscillator, which effectively varied the tuning of the band-pass analysis filter to select successive frequencies for analysis. The signal from the magnetic drum was fed into the filter, and after a sufficient number of drum revolutions a complete picture was built up, in the form of closely spaced horizontal lines of varying blackness.

Spectrographs working on this same basic principle are still in widespread use today in phonetics and other laboratories. More modern spectrographs often use digital memory to store the signal instead of analogue storage on a magnetic drum, and at least one commercially available model uses a tunable digital filter, instead of the heterodyne analysis method with an analogue filter. Although the various spectrographs and computer programs for making spectrograms differ greatly in their ease of use and in the quality of

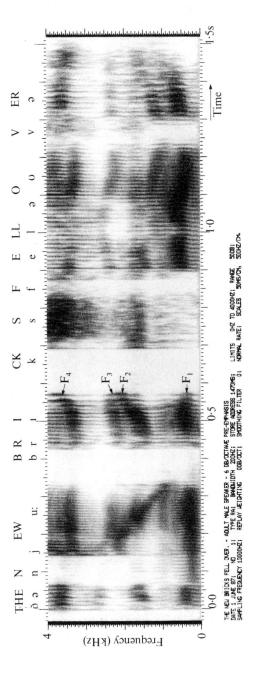

Fig. 2.10 Wide-band (200 Hz) spectrogram of the speech waveform shown in Fig. 2.9. The dynamic range of the grey scale is 50 dB, so very weak sounds are clearly visible.

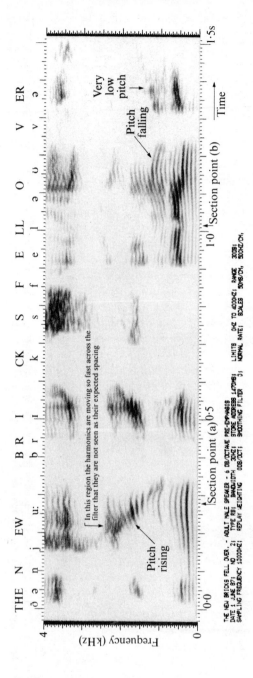

Fig. 2.11 Narrow-band (30 Hz) spectrogram of the speech waveform shown in Fig. 2.9. The dynamic range of marking in this picture in only 30 dB so weak sounds are not visible, but the harmonic structure of vowels is clearly seen.

the pictures they produce, the types of display obtained from all these methods are essentially equivalent.

One very important parameter in short-time Fourier analysis is the width (and also the shape) of the time window. A long window corresponds to a narrow band-pass filter, and if the bandwidth is appreciably less than the fundamental frequency of phonation the analysis will separate the individual harmonics of the voiced excitation source. If the time window is short it will only contain at most the response to one excitation pulse, which cannot display the harmonic structure. In effect, the bandwidth of the equivalent filter is wider than the fundamental frequency and so the harmonics will not be separated. With a wide filter, because its impulse response is shorter, the instrument will display the fine time structure of the signal in more detail than with a narrow filter. Figs 2.10 and 2.11 show wide and narrow band spectrograms of the same short sentence from a typical adult male speaker. From the wide-band spectrogram it is easy to see the formant movements, and the responses to the individual glottal excitation pulses can be seen in the time pattern of the display for each formant. On the other hand, the narrow-band picture shows the harmonic structure clearly, but blurs the rapid changes. Although the formant movements are still embodied in the variations of harmonic intensities, they are much more difficult to discern because of the distracting effect of the independent movements of the harmonics. The useful range of filter bandwidths for speech analysis lies between about 25 and 400 Hz. Narrow-band spectrum cross-sections of the marked points in Fig. 2.11 are shown in Fig. 2.12.

2.7 SPEECH PRODUCTION MODELS

If the various functions of human speech production can be modelled, either acoustically, electronically, or in a computer program, it will be possible to produce speech synthetically. Although early such attempts used acoustic models (see Linggard (1985) for a comprehensive review), electronic models took over in the 1930s, and computer models are also widely used today. In all these models the utterances to be spoken must be provided in the form of control signals that, in effect, represent the muscular control of the human vocal system. Because of the inertia of the articulators, such control signals do not change extremely fast, and can be represented well enough for almost all practical purposes within a bandwidth of 50 Hz, or by sample values every 10 ms.

For speech synthesis applications it is necessary to be able to model the sound sources, and the resonant structure of the vocal tract. The methods to be used for these two operations are not independent. If it is required to model the human speech production process very closely it should ideally be necessary to model the detailed mechanics of vocal fold vibration, and also to have models of turbulent and plosive excitation that can be inserted in the

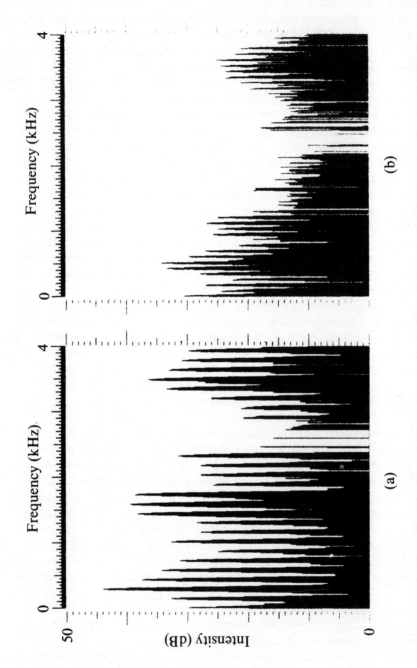

Fig. 2.12   Narrow-band spectral cross-sections, taken at the points marked on Fig. 2.11. (a) Section through the vowel in 'new'. (b) Section through the final consonant of 'fell'.

appropriate places in an articulatory model of the complete vocal tract. In principle such models are possible, but there are enormous practical difficulties in making them adequately represent realistic speech production.

2.7.1 Excitation models

Ishizaka and Flanagan (1972) modelled vocal fold vibration on a computer by considering each fold as two adjacent masses, representing the upper and lower parts, coupled by springs. They found that this model well represented the gross behaviour of real vocal folds, in that it would start and stop phonation in generally plausible ways as the sub-glottal pressure and vocal fold spacing were given appropriate values. However, this model is unable to represent the more subtle aspects of the motion of real vocal folds, such as are seen on high-speed motion pictures of the larynx. For more complicated models the computation time is greatly increased and it becomes much more difficult to deduce realistic values for the parameters of a more elaborate structure. For these reasons it is not usual to use models of the actual vocal folds in practical speech synthesis, but instead to use other means for generating some functional approximation to the voiced excitation signal.

Bearing in mind that the most important property of the glottal flow is excitation of the formants at every glottal closure, it is possible to represent the flow merely by a train of impulses repeating at the fundamental frequency. As a real glottal pulse has most of its energy at low frequencies, an impluse train, with its flat spectral envelope, will not produce the correct relative intensities of the formants. However, the spectral balance can be approximately corrected by a simple linear filter. As the ear is not very sensitive to moderate amounts of phase distortion, even using a minimum-phase filter can gave an excitation source that approximates fairly well to the important features of glottal excitation. A much better approximation, that is still much easier to generate than a vocal fold model, is achievable by representing the air-flow pulse shape by some simple mathematical function (e.g. by a small number of segments from a cosine wave). By varying the numerical parameters specifying each segment it is then even possible to model the variations in shape with vocal effort, and some of the differences between different speakers. Closer approximations to more complex pulse shapes can be produced by storing one or more typical shapes as sets of waveform samples, and repeating those sample sequences at the required fundamental frequency. To get good results by this technique it is necessary to have some method of varying the time scale of the pulses, particularly as the fundamental frequency varies.

As most speech synthesizers these days are implemented digitally, using sampled-data filters, it is naturally attractive for implementation to make voiced excitation pulses have a spacing equal to an integer number of sampling periods. At the usual sampling rates of around 10 kHz this quantization of pulse positions can cause noticeable roughness in the perceived pitch of synthetic speech, particularly for high pitches, and so it is also desirable to have some means of interpolating excitation points between the signal samples. If these precautions are taken, the stored-shape models of voiced excitation can be used to generate synthetic speech almost totally indistinguishable from high-quality recorded natural speech.

Turbulent excitation can be very well modelled by random electrical noise, or, in digitally implemented synthesizers, by a pseudo-random sequence generator. On occasions when fricative and voiced excitation is produced simultaneously, the fricative intensity in natural speech will be modulated by the periodically varying air flow through the glottis. It is not difficult to represent this effect in a synthesizer, particularly in digital implementations, although there seems little evidence so far that it influences perception of even the highest-quality synthetic speech.

Plosive excitation can be well represented by a single impulse, in conjunction with an appropriate filter to achieve the desired spectrum shape. However, as the spectral fine structure of a single pulse is the same as that of random noise, it is quite usual to use the same noise generator for plosive as for fricative excitation. The difference will be that the phase coherence of impulsive excitation will not then be achieved on plosive bursts. As the duration of such bursts normally lasts only a few milliseconds, the difference can only be perceived under very favourable listening conditions.

2.7.2 Vocal tract models

As with the vocal folds, it is also possible to make a computer model to represent the physical structure of the remainder of the vocal system. The limitations of a simple acoustic tube model have already been discussed. Some improvement can be achieved by modelling the losses distributed along the tube, and Flanagan et al. (1975) have done this by representing the vocal tract by a simulation of a 20-section lumped constant transmission line with realistic losses in each section. With their complete model, comprising the vocal folds and the simulated pharyngeal, oral and nasal tracts, they have successfully produced complete utterances by controlling dimensions and other parameters of the model to copy the articulatory behaviour of real speakers. However, the difficulties of determining and controlling the details of the model parameters are extreme, and their model does not attempt the very difficult task of representing the departures from plane wave propagation. For these reasons, although articulatory synthesis is already providing valuable insights into the mechanism of speech production, it is likely to be very many years before it will be practicable to use it for everyday generation of synthetic speech.

There is, however, a particular use of the acoustic tube model for speech synthesis which is both practical and very widely used. An acoustic tube with

N sections has N degrees of freedom in its specification (usually represented by the N reflection coefficients at the section boundaries). These N degrees of freedom are responsible for determining the N coordinates of the independent poles in its transfer function. (Each pair of poles can be complex conjugate or real, in both cases requiring two coordinates to specify two poles.) When fed with a suitable excitation signal, the dimensions of the tube can be chosen so that those poles give the best possible approximation to spectral properties of a short segment of speech signal, according to some suitable error criterion. If N is made sufficiently high, but the sampling rate of the synthesizer is kept near the Nyquist rate for the bandwidth of signal required (e.g. around 10 kHz) it is possible to make an all-pole minimum-phase filter that will give a very close approximation to any actual spectral shape of a speech signal. If N is made sufficient to represent the number of formants within the given bandwidth, and if the speech sound being produced is the result of an unbranched vocal tract excited at the glottis, then the resultant acoustic tube shape will approximate reasonably well to the area function of the vocal tract that produced the sound. In general, however, this will not be so, and some of the poles of the filter will often be real, with a role for controlling the general spectral balance of the signal instead of providing resonant modes. The analysis method used for this type of synthesizer, known as **linear predictive coding** (see Chapter 4), is not concerned with modelling the articulation, but merely with optimizing the filter specification to make the best approximation to acoustic properties of the signal. It is just an incidental property of the method that under the right conditions (i.e. for non-nasal vowels) the articulatory approximation of the equivalent tube is not too bad.

The practical alternative to articulatory synthesis is merely to generate the signal by means of excitation provided to a set of resonators for representing the individual formants. If there are, say, five formants to be modelled within the desired audio bandwidth, then five resonators will be needed. There are two basic ways in which such resonators can be connected – **cascade** or **parallel**. If they are connected in cascade (Fig. 2.13) there is only one

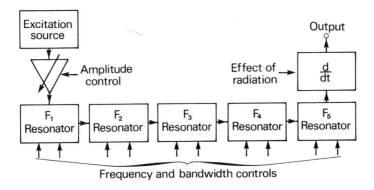

Fig. 2.13 Cascade connection of formant generators.

amplitude control, and the relative intensities of the formants are determined entirely by their frequencies and their damping factors or bandwidths. If sampled-data resonators are used, the resultant all-pole filter will be exactly equivalent to the acoustic tube model referred to in the last paragraph, except that the filter will be specified in terms of formant frequencies and bandwidths instead of tube reflection coefficients. This different method of specification has the advantage that it can be easily related to the acoustic properties of speech, as seen on spectrograms, but it will not in general be easy to model the effects of variation of vocal effort on the voiced source spectrum, of excitation inserted further forward than the glottis, or of nasal coupling. For these reasons cascade-formant synthesis in its simplest form is normally used only for modelling non-nasal vowels, and complete synthesizers using this method are usually provided with other methods for generating plosives, fricatives and nasals.

The claimed advantage of cascade formants over the parallel connection for non-nasal vowels is that it offers a theoretical representation of the unbranched acoustic tube. While this is true, a synthesizer with parallel resonators is, in fact, able to approximate just as well to the unbranched tube for all practical purposes, if sufficient care is taken over the design details.

If a small number (e.g. four or five) of analogue resonators are used to model the formants in a cascade synthesizer, the transfer function will not have the infinite series of poles that is present with sampled-data systems. The result in the speech frequency range will be to remove the combined effect of the lower skirts of the infinite number of periodic poles that the sampled-data implementation would give, so making the upper formants much less intense. When analogue cascade synthesizers were still in common use, the solution to this problem was to include a special **higher-pole correction circuit** which gave an approximation to the effect of the missing higher poles that was fairly accurate up to about 5 kHz.

With a parallel-formant synthesizer, the outputs from the separate resonators are added, and each one has its own separate gain control to vary the formant intensity. The increase in formant amplitude when two formants move close in frequency, which occurs automatically in an all-pole cascade-formant synthesizer, has to be provided explicitly in the amplitude controls of a parallel system. Thus more control information has to be provided. The transfer function of a parallel connection of resonators will have the same poles as the cascade connection, but will also in general have zeros which are a direct consequence of the parallel paths. The zero coordinates can be found by putting the second-order transfer functions of the individual resonators over a common denominator, and then factorizing the resultant numerator.

The phase characteristics of individual resonators show a change from 90° lead to 90° lag as the frequency passes resonance, and so between any pair of adjacent formants the phase characteristics will differ by approximately 180°. If the formant waveforms are combined by simple addition there will be a deep dip in the spectrum, caused by the zeros, between every pair of formants

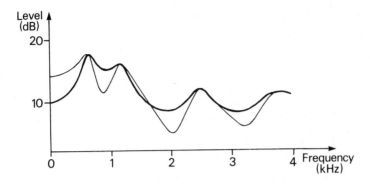

Fig. 2.14 Thick line: typical spectral envelope during a vowel. Thin line: the result of simple addition of the outputs from parallel-formant generators.

(Fig. 2.14). Such deep dips do not normally occur in the spectrum of human speech. If, on the other hand, the gain coefficients of adjacent formants have opposite signs the responses from the skirts of neighbouring formants will reinforce each other. In effect this change will move the zeros of the transfer function well away from the frequency axis in the s plane (or from the unit circle in the z plane for sampled-data synthesizers). In fact, if all resonators are arranged to have the same bandwidth, it is possible to choose the gain coefficients so that the transfer function reduces to an all-pole one, and the parallel circuit will then have the identical response to a cascade connection.

The advantage of a parallel-formant synthesizer is that it enables a reasonable approximation to be achieved for the spectral shape of sounds for which the all-pole design is not well suited. As the perceptual properties of speech are largely determined by the frequencies and intensities of the formants, it is possible to represent these properties very well by a suitable excitation signal feeding a parallel set of resonators with the appropriate frequency and amplitude parameters. In fact it is most convenient in such a system to incorporate the different spectral trends of the different types of excitation simply by varying the formant amplitude controls, so that both voiced and voiceless excitation are arranged to have the same spectral envelope. The difficulties with this method arise when formants in different parts of the spectrum are set to have very different amplitudes. During voiceless fricatives the high formants will be very intense while F_1 will be extremely weak, and the reverse will occur in nasal consonants. The skirts of the frequency responses of some resonators may then be of comparable level to the signal required at the peaks of the other, less intense, resonances. There will then be a danger that the assumptions about spectral shape between the formants will not be justified, and the overall response will not be acceptable, particularly at the very low and very high ends of the spectrum.

By putting very simple filter circuits in each formant output to modify the shape of the formant skirts before mixing, it is possible to achieve a very

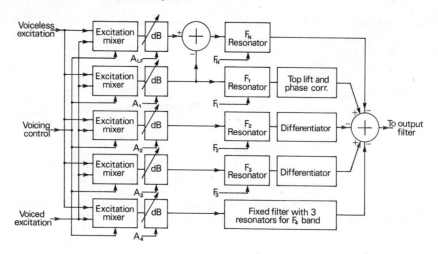

Fig. 2.15 Block diagram of the parallel-formant filter system described in Holmes (1983).

acceptable approximation to the overall spectral shape of any speech sounds using a parallel-formant synthesizer. A block diagram of a complete formant system of this type is shown in Fig. 2.15. There are two features of the spectral shape specification that deserve special comment. The first is the use of a special heavily-damped low-frequency resonator (F_N) below the frequency of F_1. By choosing the appropriate setting of A_{LF} it is possible to control the level in the bottom few hundred hertz independently of the level of F_1, to give a better control of the low-frequency spectral shape of vowels, and more particularly of nasalized vowels and nasal consonants. The second feature is the use of a fixed filter with multiple resonances in the F_4 region. Because of the cross-dimensions of the vocal tract the region above 3 kHz often has many more resonant modes than are predicted by the simple acoustic tube theory, but the detail of the spectral shape in this region is not important. The approximation given by this fixed filter, when it is supplied with the appropriate amplitude control, is perceptually completely sufficient to achieve the highest speech quality.

The excitation circuits for the synthesizer shown in Fig. 2.15 have provision for mixed voiced and voiceless sound sources. In human speech, when voiced and turbulent sources are simultaneously in operation, the lower formants will be predominantly voiced, whereas the upper formants will be predominantly voiceless. This difference arises as a direct consequence of the different spectral balance and different points of application of the two sources. The synthesizer shown in Fig. 2.15 has a separate excitation mixing circuit for each formant generator. The mixing fraction is arranged to be different for the different formants, and is controlled by an overall 'degree of voicing' signal. When the speech is half voiced the lowest formant receives only voiced excitation, the middle ones have a mixture, and the highest formant is completely voiceless. Experience has shown that this method is extremely successful in generating voiced fricatives and stops.

**SUMMARY
Chapter 2**

Models of human speech production help understanding of the nature of speech signals as well as being directly useful for speech generation.

Muscular force on the lungs provides air flow which is modulated by vibrating vocal folds in the larynx, or by turbulence or a blockage in the vocal tract. The resultant sound sources have their spectra modified by the acoustic resonances (or formants), whose frequencies are controlled by the position of the tongue, etc.

Vowels and some consonants normally use the vocal fold sound source, which is periodic with a fundamental frequency (which determines the pitch) typically in the range 50 – 400 Hz, and thus has a line spectrum. Most consonants use turbulence as the main sound source.

For many sounds the resonant structure can be approximately analysed using electrical transmission line theory by representing it as a set of acoustic tubes of different cross-section butted together. It has a transfer function which has only poles, and in spite of the idealizations in the analysis, this function gives a fairly good specification of the three or four main resonances. For most consonant sounds the simple acoustic tube analogue is not really adequate, and more complicated tube analysis is not very practical. Nasal sounds require the very complicated structure of the nose to be considered, and the way it couples with the pharynx and mouth. Other consonants normally have a close constriction in the mouth, which effectively decouples the back part of the acoustic system and makes it easier to consider only the part in front of the constriction.

During many voiced sounds the effect of the glottal impedance on the resonances of the vocal tract causes a substantial extra damping when the vocal folds are at their farthest apart.

The effect of radiation at the mouth can be well represented by simple differentiation of the volume flow waveform.
Spectrograms are generally a more useful way of dis-

playing the significant properties of speech sounds than are waveforms. Narrow-band spectrograms clearly show the change in pitch, whereas wide-band spectrograms are better for illustrating formant structure.

The speech production process can be modelled electronically, and such models are used as practical speech synthesizers. These days they are mostly implemented digitally using sampled-data techniques.

The details of vocal fold vibration need not be copied closely for realistic speech synthesis, provided the main acoustic consequences are represented. Turbulence is easily represented by random electrical noise or a pseudo-random sequence generator, and plosive excitation by a single impluse or by a very short burst of random noise.

Speech synthesis can, in principle, use vocal tract (articulatory) models for the resonant system, but these are mostly too complicated to control except for the special case of linear predictive coding (LPC, see Chapter 4). More practical models use explicit separate resonators for the formants. The resonators can be connected in cascade, which is theoretically attractive for vowels but unsuitable for most consonant sounds. When carefully designed, a parallel resonator system using individual amplitude controls can give excellent results for all types of speech sound. A realistic representation of mixed vocal fold and turbulent excitation can also be provided in a parallel-formant system.

EXERCISES
Chapter 2

E2.1 What are the main differences between the spectra of voiced and voiceless excitation?

E2.2 What are the possible contributions to voiced excitation besides air flow through the glottis?

E2.3 Discuss the idealizing assumptions that are made in the simple theory of vocal tract acoustics.

E2.4 Describe the effects of having the sound source remote from the glottis during consonant production.

E2.5 In what ways are fundamental frequency and formant frequencies interdependent?

E2.6 Give examples of factors which influence formant bandwidth.

E2.7 Why is a spectrogram more useful than the waveform when studying the communication function of speech signals?

E2.8 Discuss the different uses of wide-band and narrow-band spectrograms.

E2.9 Summarize the relative merits of cascade and parallel formant synthesis.

E2.10 Why has articulatory synthesis been less successful than formant synthesis?

3

MECHANISMS AND MODELS OF THE HUMAN AUDITORY SYSTEM

3.1 INTRODUCTION

When considering the requirements for speech synthesis, or methods for automatic speech recognition, much insight can be gained from knowledge of the workings of the human auditory system. Unfortunately, because of the invasive nature of most physiological studies and the large number and extremely small size of the neurons involved, study in this area has been extremely difficult, and our knowledge is very incomplete. Even so, over the recent decades much progress has been made, with a combination of psychophysical studies on humans, neurophysiological studies on experimental animals, and computer modelling to test plausible hypotheses.

3.2 PHYSIOLOGY OF THE OUTER AND MIDDLE EARS

Fig. 3.1 illustrates the structure of the human ear. The sound impinging on the side of the head travels down the passage known as the **auditory canal**, to reach the **eardrum**, or **tympanic membrane**. However, the external structure of the ear, known as the **pinna**, plays a significant role, as it causes high-frequency sound to be collected more effectively from in front of the head than behind, and so contributes to our ability to locate sound sources. The wavelength at low frequencies (say below 1 kHz) is so long that diffraction prevents the pinna from providing directional selectivity for these components of a complex sound.

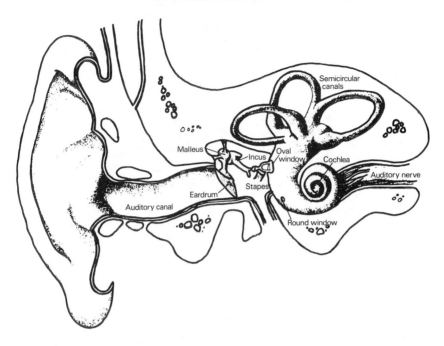

Fig. 3.1 Structure of the human auditory system. (Lindsay and Norman, 1972. Reproduced by permission of the authors).

The length of the auditory canal is such that it forms an acoustic resonator, with a rather heavily damped main resonance at about 3.5 kHz, and some slight secondary resonances at higher frequencies. The principal effect of this resonant behaviour is to increase the ear's sensitivity to sounds in the 3 – 4 kHz range.

The middle ear consists of a group of inter-connected small bones (the **ossicles,** comprising the **malleus, incus** and **stapes**) that couple the movements of the eardrum to the **oval window** at one end of the **cochlea**. The cochlea is the main structure of the inner ear. The ossicles vibrate with a lever action, and enable the small air pressure changes that vibrate the eardrum to be coupled effectively to the oval window. In this way they act as a transformer, to match the low acoustic impedance of the eardrum to the higher impedance of the input to the cochlea.

Although the pinna and the ossicles of the middle ear play a significant role in the hearing process, the main function of processing sounds is carried out within the cochlea and in higher levels of neural processing.

3.3 STRUCTURE OF THE COCHLEA

As can be seen from Fig. 3.1, the cochlea is a spiral tapered tube, with the

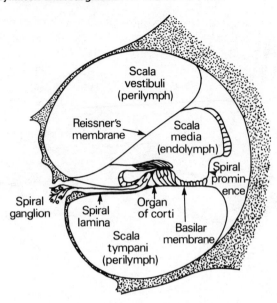

Fig. 3.2   Cross-section of one turn of the cochlear spiral.

stapes in contact with the outer, larger cross-section, end. At this end also are the **semi-circular canals**, whose main function is control of balance, rather than hearing. Fig. 3.2 shows a section through one turn of the spiral, and it can be seen that it is divided along its length into three parts by two membranes. The three parts are known as the **scala vestibuli**, the **scala media** and the **scala tympani**. The scala media is filled with a fluid known as **endolymph**. The structure separating the scala vestibuli and the scala tympani stops just short of the inner end of the cochlear spiral, to leave a small interconnecting opening known as the **helicotrema**. Both of these scalae are filled with another fluid, **perilymph**. One of the membranes, **Reissner's membrane**, is comparatively wide, and serves to separate the fluids in the scala media and the scale vestibuli but has little effect acoustically. The other membrane, the **basilar membrane**, is a vital part of the hearing process. As can be seen, the membrane itself only occupies a small proportion of the width of the partition between the scala media and the scala tympani. The remainder of the space is occupied by a bony structure, which supports the **organ of Corti** along one edge of the basilar membrane. Rather surprisingly, as the cochlea becomes narrower towards the helicotrema, the basilar membrane actually becomes wider. In humans it is typically 0.1 mm wide at the basal end, near the oval window, and is 0.5 mm wide at the apical end, near the helicotrema.

As the stapes vibrates, and so causes movements in the incompressible perilymph in the scala tympani, there are compensatory movements of the small membrane covering the **round window**, which is situated near the basal end of the scala vestibuli. If the stapes is given an impulsive movement, its immediate effect is to cause a distortion of the basal end of the basilar membrane. These initial movements are followed by a travelling wave along the cochlea, with corresponding displacements spreading along the length of the basilar membrane. However, the mechanical properties of the membrane in conjunction with its environment cause a resonance effect in the membrane movements: the different frequency components of the travelling wave are transmitted differently, and only the lowest audio frequency components of the wave cause any significant movement at the apical end.

Because of the frequency dependence of the wave motion in the cochlea it is most useful to study the response of the basilar membrane as a function of frequency, for sinusoidal stimulation. The pioneering measurements of the movement of the membrane in cadaver ears by von Békésy over 40 years ago showed a filtering action, in which each position along the membrane was associated with a frequency of maximum response. The highest audio frequencies cause most response near the basal end, and the lowest frequencies cause a peak of response near the helicotrema. However, this frequency selectivity is not symmetrical. At frequencies higher than the preferred frequency the movement falls off far more rapidly than for lower frequencies. The shape of a typical response curve as measured by von Békésy in the mid-audio range is shown in Fig. 3.3, although more recently improved measurement techniques have produced somewhat sharper curves.

For the purpose of hearing, the frequency-selective movements of the basilar membrane must be converted into a neural response. This transduction process takes place in the organ of Corti. This organ includes three rows of **outer hair cells** and one row of **inner hair cells**, which are attached to one side of the basilar membrane. The total number of hair cells in a normal human ear is nearly 30 000, spread along the cochlear spiral. Movement of the basilar membrane causes bending of the hair cells, and stimulates firing of the neurons of the auditory nerve.

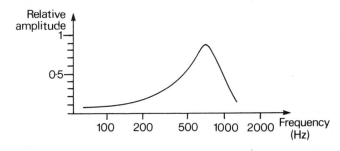

Fig. 3.3 Response of the basilar membrane as a function of frequency, measured at a point roughly a quarter of its length from the apical end. Based on data from von Békésy (1942).

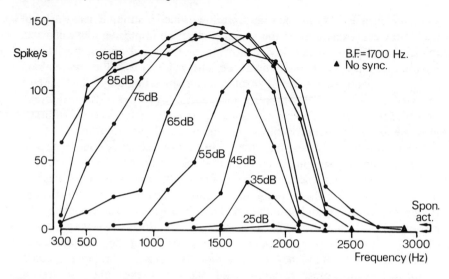

Fig. 3.4 Firing rates from a single fibre in the auditory nerve of a squirrel monkey at various intensity levels. (Rose *et al.*, 1971. Reproduced by permission of the authors).

3.4 NEURAL RESPONSE

Just as **tuning curves** can be drawn to show the mechanical movement of the basilar membrane as a function of frequency (Fig. 3.3), so it is also possible to draw curves representing the rate of firing of single nerve fibres in the auditory nerve (Fig. 3.4). It is found that each fibre has a **characteristic frequency**, at which it is most easily stimulated to fire; as might be expected, this frequency is closely related to the part of the basilar membrane associated with the corresponding hair cell. However, the neural transduction process is extremely non-linear, and so the curve shape depends very much on signal level. Most neurons show a low rate of spontaneous firing, even in the absence of stimulation, and they rarely respond at mean rates in excess of a few hundred firings per second even for very intense stimuli. Fig. 3.4 does not, of course, attempt to indicate the precise times of firing of the neurons in relation to the instantaneous value of the sinusoidal stimulus. There is a strong tendency for individual firings to be at roughly the same points on the sine wave cycle, so the 'spikes' of waveform detected on the nerve fibre show interspike intervals that are very close to integer multiples of one period of the stimulating signal. There is, however, some random timing variation around these points, such that this tendency to 'phase-locking' is no longer apparent at stimulation frequencies above about 4 kHz. There continues to be much research on the processes of neural coding of audio signals, and it is certainly not yet fully understood. However, certain facts appear to be fairly well established:

a The ability of humans to distinguish between different sounds of very high intensity is still quite good, even when the intensities of their frequency components are such that the neurons at the appropriate characteristic frequencies can be expected to be fully saturated, and firing at their maximum rate.

b The ability to distinguish changes of frequency at intensities just above the threshold of hearing is far better than could be accounted for by the selectivity of the mechanical resonance of the basilar membrane.

c The degree of phase-locking between neurons that are close on the basilar membrane increases with stimulus level, and could contribute to the ability to analyse high-level sounds.

It is known that neural systems in general have substantial cross-connection between nearby neurons, which frequently causes **lateral inhibition**, i.e. a tendency for the firing of one neuron to inhibit the firing of its neighbours. This process could be a significant part of the sharpening of the tuning curve near the auditory threshold.

3.5 PSYCHO-PHYSICAL MEASUREMENTS

In the absence of complete knowledge of the physical processes of auditory analysis, it is useful to measure the functional performance of the hearing system by means of psycho-physical experiments. In such experiments,

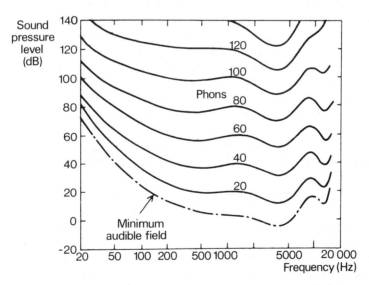

Fig. 3.5 Curves showing the sound pressure level needed for various perceived loudness values. (Robinson and Dadson, 1956. Reproduced by permission of the authors).

various types of auditory stimuli are given to human subjects, who are asked to respond in various ways according to what they hear.

One of the most basic types of auditory measurement is known as an **audiogram**, which displays the r.m.s. pressure of sound which is just audible as a function of frequency of sinusoidal stimulation. This display can be extended to include plots of subjective judgments of equal loudness at different frequencies, for levels well above the threshold of detection. Such a display is shown in Fig. 3.5. The units of loudness are **phons**, which are defined as the level in decibels of a tone at 1 kHz that would be judged to be of the same loudness as the test stimulus. The reference level for 0 dB **sound pressure level** (SPL) has been arbitrarily adopted to be 2×10^{-5} N/m^2. This level was chosen because it is approximately equal to the average threshold of hearing of humans with normal hearing at 1 kHz (which is a frequency at which our ears are nearly at their most sensitive).

On Fig. 3.5 the small ripples in auditory sensitivity in the range from 1 to 10 kHz are caused by the standing wave resonances in the auditory canal.

Perceptual experiments can be conducted to determine **psycho-physical tuning curves** (PTCs) for the auditory system. The usual method of making these measurements uses the technique of **masking**. There are many different types of masking experiment for determining the frequency resolution capabilities of the ear, of which the following is a typical example. If a low-level sinusoid (or **pure tone**) is mixed with a narrow band of random noise of much higher level and centred on the same frequency, perception of the tone will be masked by the noise. In general, the presence of the tone cannot be detected if the noise power is more than a few decibels above that of the tone. If the centre frequency of the noise is now shifted away from the tone frequency, it will not cause its main effect at the same place on the basilar membrane, and so its masking action is reduced. A PTC can be derived for any tone frequency by plotting the level of noise that is just sufficient to mask the tone, as a function of noise centre frequency. These curves can be plotted for different tone frequencies and various stimulus levels. The PTCs so derived are generally similar in form to the basilar membrane response curves (Fig. 3.3), but they are much sharper.

The useful dynamic range of representation and variation of resolution with frequency are such that it is most useful to plot PTCs with logarithmic intensity and frequency scales. The typical examples shown in Fig. 3.6 were derived by using a pure tone as the masker, and a brief low-level tone as the probe signal. The response at frequencies above the peak of sensitivity falls off at more than 80 dB/octave. The steepest slope below the peak response is nearer 40 dB/octave, but the slope then reduces to a much lower value as the frequency is further reduced. This asymmetry indicates that intense low frequencies are able to mask higher-frequency test tones much more than high frequencies will mask lower ones.

The bandwidth between 3 dB points of the PTC is around 100 Hz at low frequencies, and approximately 15% of centre frequency for higher

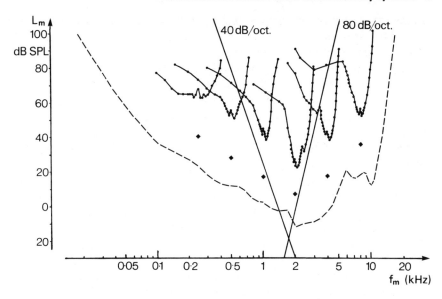

Fig. 3.6 Psycho-physical tuning curves found by a masking experiment. The dashed line shows the absolute threshold of hearing for the subject. The filled diamonds indicate the frequencies and levels of the six short probe tones that were used. The curves show the corresponding levels of masker tones needed at various frequencies to just obscure the probe tones. The superimposed sloping lines represent slopes of 40 and 80 dB/octave. (Adapted from Vogten, 1974, by permission of the author)

frequencies, above about 1 kHz. However, the estimates of bandwidth vary somewhat according to the precise experimental method used.

Because of the masking effect within the PTC bandwidth the human auditory system is not sensitive to the detailed spectral structure of a sound within this bandwidth, except to the extent that beats between spectral components cause variations of the intensity envelope that are slow enough for the neural system to respond to. The bandwidth over which the main masking effect operates is usually known as the **critical bandwidth**, but because the auditory filters do not have a rectangular response in the frequency domain, there is no very obvious way of defining the width of a critical band. One definition that has come into favour is the **equivalent rectangular bandwidth** (ERB), which is the bandwidth of an ideal rectangular pass-band filter that will transmit the same power of a flat-spectrum input as the auditory filter would, when the gains of both filters are equal at the peak-response frequency.

3.6   ANALYSIS OF SIMPLE AND COMPLEX SIGNALS

In pitch perception experiments in the mid-audio frequency range, subjects are able to perceive changes in frequency of pure tones of approximately 0.1%. It is thus clear that there is some frequency-determining mechanism that is far more powerful than the mere frequency-selective filtering of the inner ear and its associated low-level neural interactions. At frequencies above 4 kHz pitch discrimination reduces substantially. This fact gives a hint that neural phase-locking may be responsible for passing precise timing information to higher centres, so that some measurement of time intervals could be involved. Further support for some time-domain processing can be found in the ability to infer sound direction as a result of very small relative delays in signals reaching the two ears.

In the case of complex signals, such as speech, it is very much less clear what the capabilities and processes of the auditory system are. In spite of the known severe non-linearities in the relationship between neural firing and signal level, the range of SPL between signals that are just audible and those that actually cause physical discomfort is more than 100 dB (the SPL of music as produced in a modern discotheque is frequently at the upper end of this range). In the middle of the range, it is possible to vary the intensity of speech signals by at least 20 dB without listeners regarding them as being significantly changed in quality, even though they would regard these as quite substantial changes of loudness. Just discriminable differences in formant frequencies of synthetic speech signals are around 4% of their centre frequency, i.e. about 40 times less discriminable than the pitch of pure tones. There is evidence that peaks in the spectrum of the audio signal are detected more easily than features between spectral peaks, and such preferential treatment of peaks is probably caused by the shape of the PTC in combination with higher-level neural processes. By analogy with the fact that the higher levels of the visual system are known to have particular neurons that fire in response to objects of particular shape or orientation, it seems plausible that the auditory system may be able to respond specifically to formant frequency movements of particular rates, such as occur in many consonant transitions.

3.7 MODELS OF THE AUDITORY SYSTEM

Modelling of the operation of the auditory system when exposed to sound is of interest for two reasons. The first is to assist in understanding how sound is interpreted by humans and other living organisms. The second reason is to use such models directly in machines intended for processing sound that is usually interpreted by human beings – in particular for automatic speech recognition. Humans are extremely competent at interpreting speech-like sounds, even when they are modified by quite severe interfering noises or by reverberation, etc. A functional model of the auditory system might be a very good first-stage processor in a speech recognizer, because it would retain those features of a speech signal which are used for human speech recognition, but would discard information that humans make no use of.

3.7.1 Mechanical filtering

For many years people have made models of parts of the auditory system. The modelling of the outer and middle ears is fairly straightforward, at least for small or moderate sound levels, because they can then be assumed to be approximately linear and can be represented as a fairly simple electrical filter of appropriate characteristics. The main function of this filter is to model the lowest resonance of the auditory canal.

The filtering of the cochlea presents a more difficult problem. This filtering is a direct consequences of the way the waves travelling along the tapered tube interact with the mechanical properties of the basilar membrane. It is possible to represent each small section along the cochlear spiral as a section of transmission line, where the constants of each successive section are scaled to represent the narrowing of the cochlea and the changing mechanical properties of the membrane. Such models (implemented either as a lumped-constant electrical analogue or in a computer program) can be shown to yield quite close approximations to the measurements on real ears as done by von Békésy. The ability of such models to reproduce real-ear measurements gives considerable confidence that the mechanical filtering in the cochlea is now fairly well understood.

Because of the computational load involved in implementing travelling wave models in transmission lines, it is often more convenient to achieve the filtering effect merely by using a number of independent filters, each representing the filtering characteristic at a single point on the basilar membrane. Because the individual filters have a fairly broad pass-band it is possible to represent the continously distributed filter system reasonably well with as few as about 40 separate filter channels. Even with this small number the overlap between adjacent channels is so great that all significantly different filtered signals are available in at least one channel.

3.7.2 Models of neural transduction

The relationship between neural firing and basilar membrane motion is quite complicated. The saturation of firing rate at high signal levels and the phase-locking to particular points in the vibration cycle can be modelled by applying a half-wave rectification and compression function to the waveform from the auditory filter, and using the output of this process to influence the probability of firing of a model neuron. The probability of firing should, however, also be influenced by the time interval after the immediately previous firing of the same model neuron, so that a much greater stimulus will be needed to cause two firings close in time than is needed for a longer interval. To be realistic, it is also necessary to include a certain amount of randomness, to represent the fact that the time of firing of any one fibre is not precisely determined by the stimulus history. With suitable parameters for this type of model it is possible to simulate the observed firing statistics of real nerve fibres, including the slow spontaneous firing that occurs in the absence of stimulation, the saturation at high levels, and the tendency to phase-locking. By also making the firing probability depend on the average rate over the previous few tens of milliseconds it is possible to incorporate the short-term adaptation that occurs to steady sound patterns.

There have been a large number of animal studies on the responses of individual fibres in the auditory nerve. There is sufficient similarity in the physiological structure of the ears of humans and experimental animals for us to assume that the effects in human ears are very similar. There is thus a reasonable amount of confidence that the modelling of neural transduction is fairly accurate. Unfortunately it is much more difficult to get physiological data to define the further processing of these neural signals, so any modelling of the higher levels is inherently more speculative, and must be guided by the results of psycho-physical experiments.

3.7.3 Higher-level neural processing

It is clear that the average firing rate information in the auditory nerve is insufficient to account for the frequency resolution and dynamic range of the auditory system. Several workers have therefore developed models that make use of the synchrony between the firings of different neurons. When there is a peak in the input spectrum, the neural models just described will show approximately synchronous firing over a range of channels whose centre frequencies are near to the frequency of the peak. We have no clear under-standing of how real nervous systems might detect such synchrony, but functional models have been developed that seem to have the right properties.

The operation of these models uses the relationship between the interval between firings of the simulated neurons and the reciprocals of their characteristic frequencies. Models of this type have been extensively studied by, for example, Seneff (1984), who has developed **generalized synchrony detectors** (GSDs).

In Seneff's model, the signals from the neural transduction stage are assumed to represent estimates of the probability of firing of neurons connected to the corresponding parts of the basilar membrane. If there is a dominant peak in the input spectrum at the characteristic frequency of a point on the membrane, the response waveform representing the probability of firing at that point will be a half-wave rectified signal, approximately periodic at the frequency of the spectrum peak. Let this waveform be represented by $u(t)$. Let a quantity τ be defined as the reciprocal of the characteristic frequency for the neurons being considered. It follows that $u(t)$ and $u(t-\tau)$ will be very similar. For a point on the membrane slightly away from the spectrum peak, the broadly-tuned cochlear filter will still be dominated by the same spectral peak, so the periodicity of the neural response will still be the same. However, the value of τ corresponding to this point will no longer correspond to one period of the waveform, so $u(t)$ will no longer be nearly the same as $u(t-\tau)$.

$$\text{The ratio} \quad r \; = \; \frac{|u(t) + u(t-\tau)|}{|u(t) - u(t-\tau)|}$$

can be very large for points on the simulated membrane whose centre frequencies are very close to the frequency of a spectral peak, but will become much smaller for quite small movements along the membrane. The inclusion of values of u also in the numerator ensures that the peak value of r is independent of the peak magnitude of u. To avoid problems with r becoming arbitrarily large in the case of exact periodicity at a channel centre frequency, Seneff found it useful to compress the range by using the function $\arctan(r)$ as the input to her subsequent processing.

The outputs from Seneff's GSD and from similar devices developed by other workers have been found to be extremely sensitive for detecting spectral peaks associated with formants, although in the form described here they give no indication of formant intensity. Seneff was also able to make use of intensity by having her complete auditory model give an additional set of output signals depending on the mean firing rate of the simulated neurons.

Many separate research groups are currently experimenting with functional models of the properties of the higher levels of the auditory system, with many differences of detail. Some groups have already reported encouraging results from preliminary speech recognition experiments based on the use of such models.

SUMMARY
Chapter 3

The outer ear has a damped resonance which enhances the response of the tympanic membrane at around 3.5 kHz. The ossicles of the middle ear couple the vibrations of the tympanic membrane to the spiral-shaped cochlea of the inner ear.

The cochlea is filled with fluids, and divided along its length by the basilar membrane except for a small gap at the inner end of the spiral (the helicotrema). The basilar membrane shows a broadly-tuned resonant behaviour, and its resonant frequency varies along its length, being high at the outer end of the cochlea and low near the helicotrema.

Hair cells in contact with the membrane are coupled to nerve cells, and convert the membrane vibrations into neural firings in the auditory nerve. The mean rate of firing is a very non-linear function of vibration amplitude, and individual firings tend to be at a fixed part of the vibration cycle of the corresponding part of the basilar membrane.

Psycho-physical tuning curves are derived using masking techniques to show human ability to separate the responses to individual frequency components of a complex signal. Separation is not effective for components closer than a critical band, which is about 15% of centre frequency above 1 kHz and roughly constant below.

Human ability to judge the pitch of tones and the frequency of resonances is much better than indicated by the width of critical bands, and is believed to be the result of analysing the timing pattern of neural firings.

A simple filter can provide a good model of the outer and middle ears. The filtering of the cochlea can be modelled as a series of transmission line sections or as a set of discrete filters. Suitable non-linear functions applied to the filter outputs can provide estimates of the probability of neurons firing. Further processing to emulate the human ability to detect frequency changes needs to exploit the synchrony between neural firings in the outputs of the cochlear filter.

Auditory models are showing promise as acoustic analysers for automatic speech recognition.

EXERCISES
Chapter 3

E3.1 Discuss the relationship between psycho-physical tuning curves and the mechanical response of the basilar membrane as a function of frequency.

E3.2 Give possible explanations for the wide dynamic range of the human ear, given that the firing rates of individual hair cells saturate at moderate sound levels.

E3.3 Comment on the difference in frequency discrimination for simple tones and for spectral features of complex sounds, such as speech.

E3.4 Discuss the role of non-linearity in neural transduction in the ear.

E3.5 Why should it be advantageous to use models of the auditory system for speech signal analysis in automatic speech recognition?

4

DIGITAL CODING
OF SPEECH

4.1 INTRODUCTION

There are two justifications for including a chapter on speech coding in a book on speech synthesis and recognition. The first is that some specialized low data rate communication channels actually code the speech so that it can be regenerated by synthesis using a functional model of the human speaking system. The second justification arises, as will be explained in Chapter 5, because a common method of automatic speech message synthesis is to replay a sequence of message parts which have been derived directly from human utterances of the appropriate words or phrases. In any modern system of this type the message components will be stored in the machine in digitally coded form. For these reasons this chapter will briefly review some of the most important methods of coding speech digitally, and will discuss the com-promises that must be made between the number of digits that must be transmitted or stored, the complexity of the coding methods, and the intelligibility and quality of the decoded speech. Most of these coding methods were originally developed for real-time speech transmission over digital links, which imposes the need to avoid appreciable delay between the speech entering the coder and emerging from the decoder. This requirement does not apply to the use of digital coding for storing message components, and so for this application there is greater freedom to exploit variable redundancy in the signal structure.

To reproduce an arbitrary audio signal it is possible to calculate the necessary information rate (bits/s) in terms of the bandwidth of the signal and the degree of accuracy to which the signal must be specified within that bandwidth. For typical telephone quality the bandwidth is about 3 kHz and the signal/noise ratio might be 40 dB. The information rate in this case is about 40000 bits/s. For a high-fidelity monophonic sound reproducing system the bandwidth would be about five times greater, and the noise would probably be 60 – 70 dB below the peak signal level. In this case a rate of about 300000 bits/s is required to specify any of the possible distinct signals that could be reproduced by such a system.

In contrast to these very high figures, it is known that human cognitive processes cannot take account of an information rate in excess of a few tens of bits per second, thus implying a ratio of information transmitted to information used of between 1000 and 10000. This very large ratio indicates that the full information capacity of an audio channel should not be necessary for speech transmission. Unfortunately for the communications engineer, the human listener can be very selective in deciding what aspects of the signal are chosen for attention by the few tens of bits per second available for cognitive processing. Usually the listener concentrates on the message, which, with its normal high degree of linguistic redundancy, falls well within the capacity available. However, the listener may pay attention specifically to the voice quality of the speaker, the background noise, or even to the way certain speech sounds are reproduced.

There are, however, two properties of speech communication that can be heavily exploited in speech coding. The first is the restricted capacity of the human auditory system, explained in Chapter 3. Auditory limitations make the listener insensitive to various imperfections in the speech reproduction. When designing speech coding systems it can also be advantageous to make use of the fact that the signal is known to be produced by a human talker. As explained in Chapter 2, the physiology of the speaking mechanism puts strong constraints on the types of signal that can occur, and this fact can be exploited by modelling some apsects of human speech production at the receiving end of the speech link. The potential reduction in digit rate that can ultimately be achieved from this approach is much greater than is possible from exploiting auditory restrictions alone, but such systems are only suited to auditory signals that are speech-like.

In the later discussion of individual coding methods some mention will be made of the extent to which properties of perception and production are exploited. The systems presented are divided into three classes, referred to as simple waveform coders, analysis/synthesis systems and intermediate; members of each class exploit various aspects of production constraints and of perception tolerance.

4.2 SIMPLE WAVEFORM CODERS

4.2.1 Pulse code modulation

Waveform coders, as their name implies, attempt to copy the actual shape of the waveform produced by the microphone and its associated analogue circuits. If the bandwidth is limited, the **Sampling theorem** shows that it is theoretically possible to reconstruct the waveform exactly from a specification in terms of the amplitudes of regularly spaced ordinate samples taken at a frequency of at least twice the bandwidth. In its conceptually simplest form a waveform coder consists of a band-limiting filter, a sampler and a device for coding the samples. The sampler operates at a rate higher than twice the cut-off frequency of the filter. The amplitudes of the samples are then represented as a digital code (normally binary) with enough digits to specify the signal ordinates sufficiently accurately. There is obviously no point in making the specification much more accurate than can be made use of for the given input signal-to-noise ratio. This principle of coding, known as **pulse code modulation** (PCM), was suggested by Reeves (1938), and is now widely used for feeding analogue signals into computers or other digital equipment for subsequent processing (in which case it is known as **analogue-to-digital** (A–D) conversion). The process is not normally used in its simplest form for transmission or for bulk storage of speech, because the required digit rate for acceptable quality is too high. Simple PCM does not exploit any of the special properties of speech production or auditory perception expect their limited bandwidth.

The distortion caused by PCM can be considered as the addition of a signal representing the successive sample errors in the coding process. If the number of bits per sample in the code is fairly large (say > 5) this **quantizing noise** has properties not obviously related to the structure of the speech, and its effect is then subjectively equivalent to adding a small amount of flat-spectrum random noise to the signal. If the number of digits in the binary code is small or if the input signal level exceeds the permitted coder range the quantizing noise will have different properties, and will be highly correlated with the speech signal. In this case the fidelity of reproduction of the speech waveform will obviously be much worse, but the degradation will no longer sound like the addition of random noise. It will be more similar subjectively to the result of non-linear distortion of the analogue signal. Such distortion produces many intermodulation products from the main spectral components of the speech signal, but even when extremely distorted the signal usually contains sufficient of the spectral features of the original signal for much of the intelligibility to be retained.

The sound pressure waveform of a speech signal has a substantial proportion of its total power (for some speakers more than half) in the frequency range below 300 Hz, even though the information content of the signal is almost entirely carried by the spectrum above 300 Hz. As quantizing noise has a flat spectrum its effect on the signal-to-noise ratio is much more serious for the weaker but more important higher-frequency components. A considerable performance improvement for PCM can be obtained by taking into account this property of speech production, and applying **pre-emphasis** to the speech signal with a simple linear filter to make the average spectrum more nearly flat. After PCM decoding the received signal can then be restored to its original spectral shape by **de-emphasis**, so reducing the higher-frequency components of the quantizing noise. For normal communication purposes it is not, however, necessary that the de-emphasis should match the pre-emphasis, as speech intelligibility is actually improved by attenuating the low-frequency components, because it reduces the upward spread of auditory masking.

The amplitude of the quantizing noise of simple PCM is determined by the step size associated with a unit increment of the binary code. During low-level speech or silence this noise might be very noticeable, whereas during loud speech it would be masked, partially or in some cases completely, by the wanted signal. For a given subjective degradation in PCM it is therefore permissible to allow the quantizing noise to vary with signal level, so exploiting a property of perception. This variation can be achieved either by using a non-uniform distribution of quantizing levels or by making the quantizing step size change as the short-term average speech level varies. Both methods have commonly been adopted, and have enabled excellent quantizing-noise performance to be achieved at 8 bits per sample, and useful communications performance at 4 bits per sample. Civil telephony uses PCM with 8 bits per sample at 8 kHz sampling rate, so requiring 64 kbits/s. In this system there is an instantaneous **companding** characteristic that gives an approximately exponential distribution of quantizing intervals except at the lowest levels. (The two slightly different variants of this law used by different telephone administrations are known as **A-law** and **μ-law**.) The sampling rate is generous for the 300 – 3400 Hz bandwidth required, but this high sampling rate simplifies the requirements for the band-limiting filters.

The time resolution properties of the auditory system ensure that masking of quantizing noise by the higher-level wanted signals is effective for at least a few milliseconds at a time, but instantaneous companding will give finer quantization near zero crossings even for large-amplitude signals. It is obvious that more effective use will be made of the transmitted digits if the step size is not merely a function of waveform ordinate height, but is changed in sympathy with the short-term average speech level. In this case, however, some means must be devised to transmit the extra information about the quantizing step size. This information can be sent either as a small proportion of extra digits interleaved in the digital waveform description, or more usually it is embodied in the waveform code itself. The latter process is achieved by using a feedback loop in the coder that modifies the quantal step size slowly up or down according to whether the transmitted codes are near the extremities or near the centre of their permitted range. As the same codes are available at the receiver it is, in principle, easy to keep the receiver quantizing interval in step with that at the transmitter, but digital errors in the transmission path disturb this process and will thus affect the general signal level besides adding noise to the received audio waveform. Another disadvantage of this method of **backwards adaptation** is that when the signal level increases

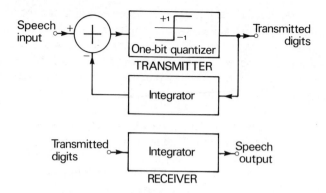

Fig. 4.1   Block diagram of a delta-modulator.

suddenly it will overload the coder for at least a few samples before the quantizing interval has had time to adapt. Use of a separate channel for **forwards adaptation** of the quantizing control can avoid this problem, but needs a small signal delay to enable the quantizer to be correctly set before the signal is coded.

4.2.2   Delta-modulation

Delta-modulation is a widely used alternative type of waveform coding. A delta-modulator uses its transmitted digital codes to generate a local copy of the input waveform, and chooses successive digital codes so that the copy reproduces the input waveform as closely as possible, within the constraints of the coding scheme. The basic scheme is illustrated in Fig. 4.1. In its original and simplest form the quantizer uses only one bit per sample, and merely indicates whether the copy is to be increased or decreased by one quantum. Such a coder offers the possibility of extremely simple hardware implement- ation, and if run at a high enough sampling rate can approximate waveforms very closely. The process of following the waveform in small steps makes delta-modulation work best on signals in which differences between successive ordinates are small. Thus the low-frequency dominance in speech signals is accommodated directly by delta-modulation without pre-emphasis, and it is acceptable to use a quantal step that is only a very small fraction of the waveform amplitude range. In contrast, a flat-spectrum input would cause frequent **slope overloading** if used with the same step size and sampling rate. Typical waveforms in simple delta-modulation are illustrated by Fig. 4.2

The use of a single bit per sample in delta-modulation is basically inefficient because a sampling rate much in excess of twice the highest frequency in the input signal is needed for close following of the input waveform. However, the intrinsic feedback loop in the waveform coding process gives the coder

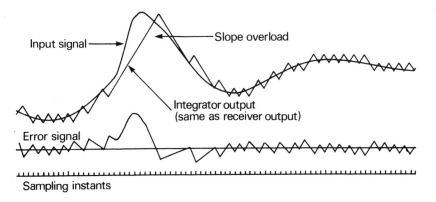

Fig. 4.2 Waveforms in a simple delta-modulator.

some 'memory' of coding overload on previous waveform ordinates, for which it continues to compensate on later samples. This advantage of delta-modulation can be combined with those of PCM if a PCM coder is used instead of a one-bit quantizer in the feedback loop. Current terminology describes this arrangement as **differential PCM** (DPCM).

The advantages of and techniques for level adaptation apply to delta-modulation in the same way as to PCM, and adaptive forms of coder are normally used, so exploiting the noise masking properties of auditory perception and the slow level changes of speech production. Adaptive DPCM (ADPCM) seems to be the most efficient of the straightforward waveform coding processes. At 16 kbits/s the quantizing noise is noticeable, but slightly less objectionable than the noise given by adaptive delta-modulation or adaptive PCM at the same digit rate. At 32 kbits/s ADPCM can give good quality speech of telephone bandwidth. This 32 kbits/s ADPCM should not be confused with the recent CCITT standard in which the term ADPCM has been extended to include systems in which the simple integrator of traditional DPCM is replaced by a higher-order backwards-adaptive filter. Because of its higher complexity, this latter technique is considered in the intermediate category (section 4.4).

4.3 ANALYSIS/SYNTHESIS SYSTEMS (VOCODERS)

The **vocoder** (a contraction of VOice CODER) was first described by Dudley of Bell Telephone Laboratories (1939). It is based on a model of speech production which exploits the fact that it is possible substantially to separate the operations of sound generation and subsequent spectrum shaping. The basic elements of a vocoder are shown in Fig. 4.3. The sources of sound are modelled by periodic or random excitation (in some vocoders mixtures of the two are also permitted). This excitation is used as the input to a dynamically

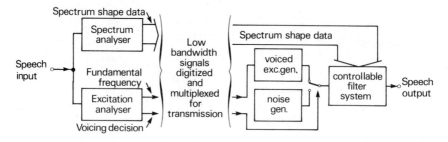

Fig. 4.3   Block diagram of the basic elements of a vocoder.

controllable filter system. The filter system models the combined effects of the spectral trend of the original sound source and the frequency response of the vocal tract. The specifications for the sound sources and for the spectral envelope are both derived by analysis of the input speech. By separating the fine structure specification of the sound sources from the overall spectral envelope description, and specifying both in terms of a fairly small number of slowly varying parameters, it is possible to produce a reasonably adequate description of the speech at data rates of 1000 – 3000 bits/s. The general principles of synthesis used in the receiver to regenerate speech from this description are discussed in section 2.7.

The important differences in principle between different types of vocoder are in the means of specifying the variable spectral shaping filter. Although many types have been demonstrated in research studies, there are currently three types of vocoder of much greater importance than any others. These are known as **channel vocoders, linear predictive coding** (LPC) **vocoders** and **formant vocoders**. With all these types the data are coded into **frames** associated with speech spectra measured at intervals of 10 – 30 ms.

Overall the advantages and disadvantages of LPC and channel vocoders are nearly equally balanced; both give usable but rather poor speech transmission performance at 2400 bits/s using fairly complex equipment. The advent of digital signal processing chips had made implementation much easier, and standard LPC is somewhat simpler than a channel vocoder when these devices are used. There are special advantages and problems with formant vocoders, and their implementation is much more complex, as explained in section 4.3.3.

4.3.1 Channel vocoders

In a channel vocoder (of which Dudley's was the first example) the spectrum is represented by the response of a bank of contiguous variable-gain band-pass filters. The way the desired overall response can be approximated using the separate contributions from individual channels is shown in Fig. 4.4. The

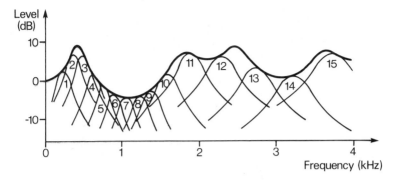

Fig. 4.4 Contributions of individual channels to a channel vocoder output spectrum. Thick line: desired spectrum shape. Thin lines: contributions from the separate channels.

control signals for the channels are derived by measuring the short-term average power from a similar set of filters fed with the input speech signal in the transmitter.

Unless a very large number of channels can be used (with consequent high digit rate) it is difficult to achieve a good approximation to the spectrum shapes around the formant peaks with a channel vocoder. However, the quality achievable with around 15 – 20 channels is reasonably acceptable for communications purposes, and does not require too high a data rate for transmission.

4.3.2 LPC vocoders

In LPC vocoders the spectral approximation is given by the response of a sampled-data filter, whose all-pole transfer function is derived from the filter that gives a least-squared error in waveform prediction, as explained below. The configuration of such a filter is illustrated in Fig. 4.5, which also indicates how the same type of filter system is used for adaptive predictive coding (see section 4.4.3).

The principle of linear prediction applied to a resonant system depends on the fact that resonance causes the future output of a system to depend on its previous history, because resonant modes continue to 'ring' after their excitation has ceased. The characteristics of this ringing are determined by a linear differential equation of appropriate order (or a difference equation in a system using sampled data). If a system is ringing entirely as a result of previous excitation, and can be represented exactly by a small number of resonant modes with constant characteristics, a difference equation can be derived to predict its future output exactly. In speech, however, these assumptions are only approximately true. Although the formants cause a

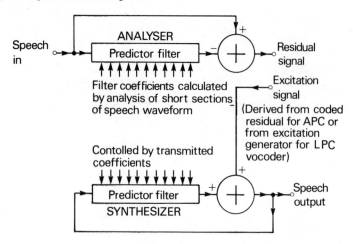

Fig. 4.5 Predictor filter as used in LPC and APC systems. When connected as shown in the synthesizer, the finite-impulse-response predictor filter provides the feedback path in an all-pole recursive filter.

strong resonance effect, they vary slowly with time. Their damping is also modified by opening and closing of the glottis. The resonances are always being excited to some extent by the sound sources, and receive substantial excitation at the instants of glottal closure. In spite of all these deviations from the ideal, it is possible to derive a useful description of the spectrum by optimizing the parameters of a predictor filter to minimize the average prediction error power over a 'frame' of input samples of around 10–20 ms duration. The predictor characteristics so obtained can then be used to resynthesize the corresponding frame at the receiver. The two main methods that are used for optimization are known as the **covariance** and **auto-correlation** methods, but their details are outside the scope of this book.

When the predictor filter has been adjusted to predict the input as best it can from the immediately preceding samples, the error signal (known as the **residual**) will have a roughly flat spectrum, and the obvious spectral peaks caused by the resonances of speech production will have been removed. For this reason the complete filtering process is sometimes referred to as **inverse filtering.**

In LPC vocoders the resonant properties of the synthesis filter make possible fairly good approximations to the spectral shapes of the formants. However, the correct analysis to achieve this result will only be obtained when the overall speech spectrum really is like the response of an all-pole filter. During vowel sounds this approximation is often very close, although at normal frame rates LPC cannot deal correctly with the fact that the formant bandwidths in natural speech change significantly as the glottis opens and closes in each excitation period. There are frequent other occasions when the spectral modelling is quite poor, particularly during nasalized vowels and

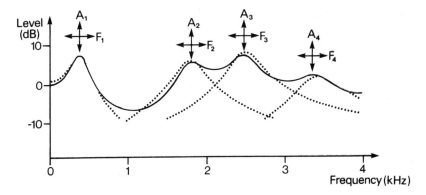

Fig. 4.6 Illustration of how formant amplitude and frequency control signals affect the output spectrum in a formant vocoder. Thick line: desired spectrum. Dotted line: contributions from individual formants.

many voiced consonant sounds. On these occasions the LPC synthesis frequently produces spectral peaks whose bandwidths are too large, with a consequent 'buzziness' in the speech quality. Another inherent property of normal LPC vocoders is that all regions of the spectrum are treated equally with regard to accuracy of frequency specifications, and so no advantage is taken of the variable frequency resolution of auditory perception.

4.3.3 Formant vocoders

In formant vocoders the spectrum is specified in terms of the frequencies and amplitudes associated with the resonant modes of the speaker's vocal tract. The relationship between the formant control signals and the synthesized spectral shape can be seen from Fig. 4.6.

Formant vocoders are very different from the channel and LPC types. They use a synthesizer that is much more closely related to human speech production, because not only do they use the choice of periodic or noise sources as in other vocoders, but also the spectral filter system has resonators that are explicitly related to the principal formants of the input speech. Thus the coding system can be constrained to deal only with the known frequency range and necessary accuracy of specification of each formant. The systematic variation of formant bandwidth with glottal opening can easily be provided in a formant synthesizer and requires no extra transmitted information. Apart from this effect, the bandwidths of the formants do not vary much during speech and such variation as does occur is fairly predictable; provided they are within the limits of natural variation, preservation of the actual formant bandwidths is not perceptually important. In consequence this property of the resonances is not normally transmitted in formant vocoders. For formant vocoders it is not practicable to use a simple cascade connection of resonators (Fig. 2.13), because occasional errors of formant frequency would then also cause serious formant amplitude errors. The parallel connection, such as is shown in Fig. 2.15, is therefore necessary.

Analysis is the main difficulty with formant vocoders. When the spectral envelope of a speech sound shows a small number of well-defined peaks it is trivial to assign these to formants in a sensible way. However, there are occasions, particularly in consonants, near vowel/consonant boundaries or even in the middle of vowels if the fundamental frequency is very high, when it is not clear what is the most appropriate way to assign the parameters of the synthesizer to spectral peaks of the input signal. Because of the analysis difficulties no formant vocoders have yet been used operationally, but a few have been demonstrated in a research environment, and some of these have been extremely successful, though computationally expensive. Formant analysers have been used to derive stored components for message synthesis, because the analysis can then be done more slowly than real time on only a moderate amount of speech material, and serious analysis errors can be corrected by subsequent interactive editing. This possibility is, of course, not available for real-time conversation.

4.3.4 Efficient parameter coding

For all types of analysis/synthesis system it is possible to achieve some saving in digit rate by exploiting the redundancy in the measured parameters. With modern implementation technology it is possible to do quite complicated coding in single-chip microprocessors, and the designer is greatly assisted by the fact that the analysis process itself gives such a reduction of digit rate compared with the original speech that the computational speed needed for further processing may be quite small for many types of coding algorithm. One obvious type of coding considers only one frame at a time, and exploits the fact that the multi-dimensional parameter space is not uniformly occupied. **Vector quantization** is a technique for selecting from a subset of possible combinations of parameter values; it requires less bits per frame than independent coding of the parameters, but it can be computationally expensive to derive the maximum benefit that is, in principle, possible with this technique.

It is also possible to make a reduction in data rate by taking into account the relationship between the data in a sequence of frames, although it will always be necessary to provide buffer delay for this reduction to be exploited in a constant-rate real-time link. In its simplest form the process can consist of merely repeating the previous frame if it is similar enough to the current one. More elaborate schemes for interpolating between selected frames some distance apart in time are also possible, and are most suited to formant vocoders because the control parameters tend to vary in a much more orderly way then they do in either channel or LPC vocoders. Such schemes appear to have the potential to achieve very good speech quality for real-time systems at about 1200 bits/s. Lower rates are possible for coding stored message components, because variable-rate coding is acceptable and interactive editing is possible to overcome some of the limitations of automatic coding.

4.4 INTERMEDIATE SYSTEMS

There are many ways of combining some of the detailed signal description possibilities of simple waveform coders with some of the signal redundancy exploitation of vocoders. The resultant intermediate systems normally give better speech reproduction in the 4 – 16 kbits/s range than is possible with either of the other two classes of system at these digit rates. Their complexity is, of course, always greater than for simple waveform coders, and some of the higher performance systems may be more complicated than vocoders.

4.4.1 Sub-band coding

Waveform coding can make use of masking effects and the ear's tolerance to less accurate signal specification at higher frequencies by filtering the speech signal into many bands and coding each band separately (Fig. 4.7). Systems that use this technique are known as sub-band coders. Each sub-band is coded by a waveform coding process, using a sampling rate equal to twice the bandwidth in each case. If the bands are made as narrow as the ear's critical bands the quantizing noise in each band can be largely masked by the speech

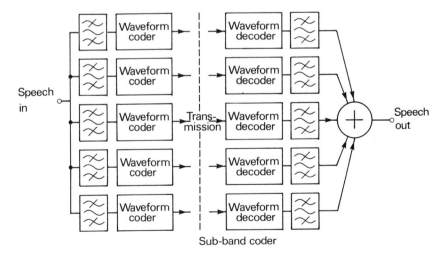

Fig. 4.7 Illustrating the principles of a sub-band coder.

signal in the same band. In addition, the fact that most power in the higher bands is from the 'unvoiced' randomly excited sounds means that the waveform shape in the these bands need not be specified so accurately, and therefore requires fewer bits per sample. In practice, complexity of suitable filter designs makes a choice of about five bands more attractive than the 15 – 20 needed for critical bands, and even with this number the speech quality in the 16 – 32 kbits/s range is much improved over that possible with the best conventional waveform coders at the same bit rates.

4.4.2 Adaptive transform coding

A different approach that utilizes both the ear's tolerance and some aspects of speech production is adaptive transform coding (ATC). The most usual implementation of this method splits the sampled speech waveform into successive blocks of 128 – 256 samples, and takes a discrete cosine transform of each block. Allocation of bits to code the transformed data can be decided adaptively for each block; by careful choice of the bit allocation it is possible to get a subjectively very close approximation to telephone speech with 16 kbits/s, and useful communication quality with only 9.6 kbits/s.

4.4.3 Methods based on linear prediction

The technique of linear prediction analysis for vocoders inherently makes available in the analyser the low-power prediction error signal. If applied as input to the LPC vocoder synthesis filter, this residual signal will regenerate the original speech waveform exactly. This fact can be exploited to give an improvement in speech quality by transmitting to the receiver a digitally coded representation of the residual to replace the conventional vocoder excitation. A further stage of prediction can be included to predict the periodicity at the fundamental frequency of excitation for voiced sounds, and the residual will then be of even lower power and will be much more random in structure. Although the residual must inherently contain important detail in its time structure, its gross spectral shape will always be fairly flat because it is the output of the LPC 'inverse filter'. The objective in coding the residual is to retain as much as possible of its perceptually important features, because the quality of the output speech will depend on the extent to which these features are available at the receiver.

There is a whole family of related techniques that all depend on linear prediction analysis, with some form of excitation derived from the residual. At one extreme is, of course, the LPC vocoder, where the excitation is generated taking into account only the periodicity of the residual, which is transmitted as a low data rate parameter. Another technique is to transmit the low-frequency waveform structure of the residual, sampled at a reduced rate,

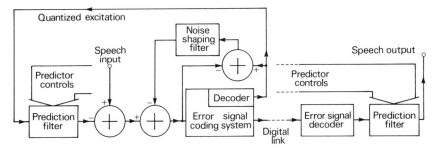

Fig. 4.8   General APC-type coder and decoder.

and to regenerate a wide-band excitation by non-linear action or by spectral folding. This method has usually been called residual-excited linear prediction (RELP). It exploits the fact that the detail of the spectrum structure is subjectively not so important at the higher audio frequencies.

Adaptive predictive coding

There is another group of techniques, of which the basic form is known as adaptive predictive coding (APC), which is illustrated in Fig. 4.8. The important features of this group are:

a They are essentially waveform coders, in that they have a feedback loop that attempts to copy the input waveform, using a suitable error criterion.

b The predictor in the feedback loop is controlled by the quantized predictor coefficients, and the quantizer used to code the residual is also placed in the feedback loop. As a result, the waveform of the residual takes into account the imperfections of both quantizers. The overall coding accuracy can then be much better than would be possible by using the same number of bits to code the residual in isolation.

c The minimization of the overall quantizing noise is done through a **noise-shaping filter** that gives less weight to the noise in the high-level regions of the spectrum. The action of the noise-shaping filter results in an increase in the total noise power, but the noise is concentrated in regions of the spectrum where the speech power is high and the noise is therefore more effectively masked by the speech signal. Comparatively more weight is given to the error signal in the low-level regions between the formants, so getting a better signal-to-noise ratio in these regions than would otherwise be achieved.

APC coders can be made either with or without a fundamental period predictor. If it is included it can have just one tap-weight, whose delay will be set to the number of samples nearest to the estimated period, or it can have a group of two or three taps on consecutive sample delays, whose weights are adjusted to minimize the residual. In the latter case it is possible to represent the fundamental periodicity even if it is not at an exact multiple of the sampling period. If the fundamental-period predictor is included the residual power will be very low during long periodic sounds, but there will still be higher-level transients whenever either the fundamental frequency or the formant frequencies change. As the ear is in general less sensitive to noise and distortion in transient sounds, the presence of this extra stage of prediction is just what is wanted to make the coding more accurate when it matters most. It is therefore always worth putting in the fundamental predictor if the extra complexity is acceptable. Only a moderate amount of extra information is needed to describe the extra filter taps, and even on completely aperiodic sounds the extra taps should not make the performance any worse.

Multipulse LPC

There are many techniques for coding the residual in the APC family of systems, and some have attained such importance that they have been given their own separate names. One of these is multipulse LPC, where the residual is represented by a much smaller number of pulses than is indicated by the Nyquist rate for the signal. 'Analysis by synthesis' is used to optimize the amplitudes and positions of these pulses to minimize the spectrally shaped quantizing noise, and it is these amplitudes and positions that are coded for transmission. Typically only 10 – 20 pulses are used for every 20 ms of speech, so reducing the sampling rate of the residual by a factor of more than 10. The success of multipulse LPC is fairly easy to understand, and stems directly from the fact that voiced speech is typically excited by only a small number of glottal pulses every 20 ms. The multipulse algorithm will place the largest excitation pulses to correspond with the main glottal excitation points, and will then add extra smaller pulses to correct for the inadequacy of the LPC filter in predicting the waveform detail. The inadequacy arises from the fact that neither the excitation nor the vocal tract response can be accurately represented by the simple models that are assumed in LPC vocoders.

Code-excited linear prediction

Another recent variant of APC has been called **code-excited linear prediction** (CELP). Demonstrations have shown excellent quality telephone bandwidth speech using only 2 kbits/s for the residual, equivalent to about 4.8 kbits/s gross. The principle is to have a set of waveform code sequences, say 1024, selected by a 10-bit code. These sequences correspond to a section of waveform of, perhaps, 40 samples, thus involving only one quarter of a bit per sample of coded residual. For each 40-sample section of residual, the available codes are tested to choose the one that minimizes the weighted quantizing error power, just as in conventional APC. At first sight one might expect this method would be critically dependent on having a very carefully chosen set of 1024 codes to represent possible residual patterns, but in fact it has been found that excellent subjective performance can be obtained by using a set of random noise sequences for the codes.

Backwards adaptive prediction

APC systems are capable of achieving very good reproduction of the input signal with less than 10 kbits/s for coding the residual, and they derive their predictor coefficients from analysis of the input signal. It is deceptively attractive to envisage that an almost equivalent performance might be obtained if the predictor coefficients were derived at the transmitter from the predicted speech waveform, which is the same as the reconstructed speech waveform that is produced at the receiver. With such a system the residual quantizer would try to make the reconstructed waveform copy the input, using the current specification of the predictor, and the predictor would be updated from an analysis of the copy waveform instead of from the input speech. As the only information used in generating the copy is the quantized residual, which is available at the receiver, it is not then necessary to transmit the predictor parameters explicitly. With such a system it is only possible to base the predictor on samples that have already been transmitted, so the prediction cannot be as accurate in rapidly changing sounds as in a frame-based system that permits a small delay in the signal. In principle the method will work, but only if it can be guaranteed that the digit streams used for deducing the predictor filter are *identical* for all time in both coder and decoder, and that the initial conditions are also identical. An error of only a single digit in the transmission will cause such a system to go unstable. Of coure, perfect accuracy of the digit stream is never guaranteed for any real communication link, but might be achievable in a computer-based message storage system. With a lower-order predictor it is possible to use this technique even for transmission if the adaptation is carefully controlled; occasional transmission errors do not then cause the system to go unstable, but the predictor is not able to give such a low residual power as is normal in APC systems. The method can be regarded as an extension to adaptive differential PCM, where the integrator (zero-order predictor) is replaced by a low-order adaptive linear predictor. The term ADPCM has been adopted to describe backwards adaptive prediction of this type, normally running at 32 kbits/s. At this rate it can give excellent quality telephone bandwidth speech. For civil telephony the CCITT (which sets telephone standards inter-nationally) has recently adopted a standard algorithm for ADPCM at 32 kbits/s that gives very little degradation to telephone-bandwidth signals.

4.5 CHOOSING A CODER

It can be seen that there is a bewildering variety of speech coding methods available, each with its own particular advantages and disadvantages, and it is very difficult for a system designer to make the best compromise between the conflicting factors which should influence the choice. Characteristics such as cost, size, weight and digit rate can be assessed using mainly engineering and economic criteria. Although such assessments are not simple, the more difficult problem is to assess how faults in the reproduction of the transmitted speech affect the human listeners. Mathematical calculations of such quantities as signal-to-noise ratio, although useful for comparing two systems of similar type, are not reliable for assessing the reaction of listeners. The ultimate criterion for judging the performance of any speech transmission or reproduction system must be the satisfaction of the human users, and properly controlled subjective testing is always necessary to ensure making the correct choice.

SUMMARY
Chapter 4

Some low data rate methods of coding for speech transmission include a speech synthesizer, and many types of digital coding are used for storing sections of natural speech for message synthesis. Speech coding always involves a three-way compromise between data rate, speech quality and equipment complexity.

Simple waveform coders, using pulse code modulation or delta-modulation, can achieve fairly good quality with very simple equipment, but require a high data rate. Adaptation of the quantizer in these coders improves the performance at any data rate with only a small increase in complexity.

Analysis/synthesis systems (vocoders) provide much lower data rates by using a functional model of the human speaking mechanism at the receiver. The excitation properties and spectral envelope are specified separately. The three main types of vocoder describe the slowly varying spectral envelope in different ways. The channel vocoder specifies the power in a set of contiguous fixed band-pass filters. LPC vocoders use an all-pole sampled-data filter to model the short-term speech spectrum. Formant vocoders specify the frequencies and intensities of the lowest-frequency formants.

Real-time speech communication of reasonable quality is possible at 2400 bits/s using either channel or LPC vocoders. Formant vocoders have potential for lower data rates, but they are not yet practicable for real-time communication.

There are also intermediate systems, that have some of the advantages of vocoders and of simple waveform coders, and often use digit rates in the 4 – 16 kbits/s range.

Many intermediate systems use linear prediction analysis to exploit the resonant properties of speech production, but with different ways of coding the prediction residual for use as excitation in the receiver. Adaptive predictive coding, multipulse linear prediction and code-excited linear prediction can all give excellent speech quality at data rates well below 16 kbits/s.

Backwards adaptive prediction, commonly referred to as adaptive differential pulse code modulation (ADPCM), has become a high-quality standard for telephone communication at 32 kbits/s.

EXERCISES
Chapter 4

E4.1 Why are simple speech waveform coders extravagant with digit rate, and why should economies be possible?

E4.2 Why is it not useful to specify the ratio of signal to quantizing noise as a performance criterion for PCM when there are very few bits per sample?

E4.3 Why are simple waveform coders greatly improved by some form of adaptation to variations in speech level?

E4.4 What are the essential features of a vocoder?

E4.5 Why do the theoretically attractive features of LPC vocoders often not result in improved performance over channel vocoders?

E4.6 Describe various possibilities for reducing the transmission data rate in vocoders.

E4.7 Discuss the role of linear prediction in various intermediate-rate coding techniques.

5

MESSAGE SYNTHESIS FROM STORED HUMAN SPEECH COMPONENTS

5.1 INTRODUCTION

Several years ago the term 'speech synthesis' was used almost exclusively for the process of generating speech sounds completely artificially in a machine which to some extent modelled the human speaking system, as described in Chapter 2. The applications were mainly for research in speech production and perception. These days, particularly in an engineering environment, speech synthesis has come to mean provision of information in the form of speech from a machine, in which the messages are structured dynamically to suit the particular circumstances required. The applications include simple information services, reading machines for the blind and communication aids for people with speech disorders. Speech synthesis can also be an important part of complicated man–machine systems, in which various types of structured dialogue can be made using voice output, with either automatic speech recognition or key pressing for the man-to-machine direction of communication.

5.2 WAVEFORM CONCATENATION

An obvious way of producing speech messages by machine is to have recordings of a human being speaking all the various words, and to replay the recordings at the required times to compose the messages. The first significant application for this technique was a speaking clock, introduced into the UK

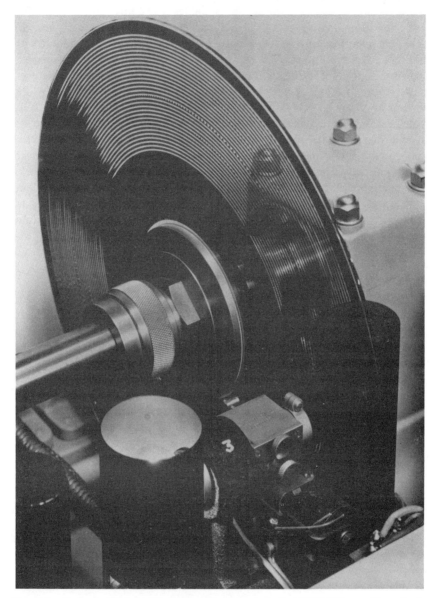

Fig. 5.1 A glass disc used for message storage in the 1936 UK speaking clock. *Courtesy of British Telecommunications plc.*

telephone system in 1936, and now provided by telephone administrations all over the world. The original UK Speaking Clock used optical recording on glass discs for the various phrases, words and part-words that were required to make up the full range of time announcements (see Fig. 5.1). Some words can be split into parts for this application, because, for example, the same recording can be used for the second syllables of 'twenty', 'thirty', etc. The next generation of equipment used analogue storage on magnetic drums. For more general applications of voice output there is a serious disadvantage with analogue storage on tapes, discs or drums: the words can only start when the recording medium is in the right position, so messages need to be structured to use words at regular intervals if delays approaching the duration of one word or more are to be avoided. If the desired messages can be successfully made merely by replaying separately stored words in a specified order, the use of recorded natural speech means that the technical quality of the reproduction can be extremely high. It is apparent from the excellent speech from speaking clocks that there are applications where this method works extremely well. In the late 1960s it was used for some announcing machine applications in association with general-purpose computers, such as to provide share prices from the New York Stock Exchange to telephone enquirers.

The development of large, cheap computer memories has made it practicable to store speech signals in digitally coded form for use with computer-controlled replay, and, provided sufficiently fast memory access is available, this arrangement overcomes the timing problems of analogue waveform storage. Digitally coded waveforms of speech signals of adequate quality for announcing machines generally use digit rates of 16–32 kbits per second of message stored, so quite a large memory is needed if many different elements are required to make up the messages.

There are now many computer voice response systems commercially available that work on the principle of stored digitally coded message elements derived from human speech. They can work well when the messages are in the form of a list, such as a simple digit sequence, or where each message unit always occurs in the same place in a sentence, so that it is comparatively easy to ensure that it is spoken with a suitable timing and pitch pattern. Where a particular sentence structure is required, but with alternative words at particular places in the sentence, it is important that the alternative words should be recorded as part of the right sort of sentence, because they would otherwise not fit in with the required sentence intonation. For list structures it is desirable to record two versions of every element that can occur either in final or non-final position. The appropriate falling pitch can then be used for the final element in each list. Even for messages that are suitable for stored waveform concatenation, great care has to be taken in recording and editing the separate message components, so that they sound reasonably fluent when presented in sequence. For any large body of messages it is worthwhile to provide a special interactive editing system, in which any section of waveform can be marked and replayed, either in isolation or joined to other sections. By this means it is possible to select the best available recording and choose the precise cutting points for greatest fluency. Even with these special tools the editing is very labour-intensive, and can take many man-months to achieve good results with a message set of moderate size.

In spite of its success for quite advanced applications, there are a number of disadvantages with using stored speech waveforms for voice output. In normal human speech the words join together, and the inherently slow movements of the articulators mean that the ends of words interact to modify the sound pattern in a way that depends on the neighbouring sounds. The pitch of the voice normally changes smoothly, and intonation is very important in achieving fluency and naturalness of speech. It therefore follows that if single versions of each word are stored they cannot produce fluent speech if joined together in the arbitrary orders that might be needed for a wide variety of messages. Over 20 years ago laboratory experiments with arbitrary messages generated in this way demonstrated that the completely wrong rhythm and intonation made such messages extremely difficult to listen to, even though the quality of the individual words was very high.

Another problem with waveform storage is merely the size of memory needed to store a large vocabulary, although the current trend in memory costs is making this disadvantage less serious. In addition there is an insuperable limitation with all systems using stored human speech in words or larger units: every message component must have been previously spoken by a human speaker. It is thus not possible to add even a single new word without making a new recording. This process requires a suitable acoustic environment and either finding the original talker to say the new material or re-recording and editing the entire vocabulary with a new talker. This restriction prevents waveform storage from giving good results in any cases where it is necessary to add new items locally to a system already in service.

5.3 CONCATENATION OF VOCODED WORDS

The large amount of digital storage needed for speech waveforms can be greatly reduced by using a low bit rate coding method for the message elements. Some ingenious methods have been developed to reduce the digit rate of stored waveforms, by exploiting various forms of redundancy. A widespread technique is to use some type of vocoder (a channel vocoder, LPC vocoder or formant vocoder, see Chapter 4), which can reduce the digit rate of the stored utterances to 2400 or even 1200 bits/s, albeit with some reduction in speech quality compared with the high digit rate stored waveform approach. A good example of the use of LPC vocoder methods to reduce the memory requirements is in the mass-produced 'Speak 'n' Spell' educational toy of Texas Instruments. Since the first introduction of single-chip LPC synthesizers in 'Speak 'n' Spell' in the late 1970s, devices of this type have become widely used for message synthesis, and many manufacturers are now offering speech synthesis products based on LPC vocoder storage.

Besides memory size reduction there is another great potential advantage with vocoder storage of message elements: the pitch and timing of messages can easily be changed without disturbing the spectral envelope pattern of the stored words. It is thus possible, in principle, to modify the prosody to suit a word's function in a sentence, without storing alternative versions of each word. The pitch is changed merely by varying the fundamental frequency parameter fed into the synthesizer, to make it different from that which was measured from the original speech. The timing can be varied by omitting or repeating occasional frames of the control data. There are, of course, difficulties in deriving suitable methods to control the timing and intonation patterns. If there is a fixed sentence structure that sometimes requires different words in particular places, the intonation pattern can be specified in advance, and merely imposed on the words that are chosen. If the sentence structures of the messages are not determined in advance it is necessary to derive the pitch and timing according to a set of rules. This aspect will be discussed in Chapter 6. Even when an appropriate prosody can be imposed, there are still problems at word boundaries because speech properties will in general not match where words join, but the results will be much more fluent than concatenated stored waveforms. Co-articulation at word boundaries can be crudely simulated with concatenation of vocoder words by applying some smoothing to the control signals where the words join. A smoothing time constant of about 50 ms will remove the more serious effects of discontinuity at the word boundaries. Alternatively, one can have an overlap region, where the parameters for the end of one word can be gradually blended with those for the beginning of the next. Such crude methods will, of course, be very unrepresentative of the actual co-articulation that occurs between words of human speech.

5.4 CONCATENATION OF SUB-WORD UNITS

The vocabulary size for word concatenation systems is limited by memory availability and by the problem of recording and editing all the words. One obvious way of overcoming this difficulty is to reduce the size of the stored units. Harris (1953) described some experiments with 'building blocks of speech', in which he tried to synthesize words by concatenating waveform recordings of the length of individual phones. He found it was essential to have several allophones of most phonemes, and even then intelligibility of some words was poor. By using waveform segments, Harris had the extra problems of pitch discontinuity. These days some low-cost synthesis products use allophone concatenation of LPC vocoder parameters, which overcomes some of the difficulties of Harris's method, but the lack of any representation of the co-articulation prevents these methods from achieving high intelligibility.

One way of using small units, while still achieving natural co-articulation, is to make the units include the transition regions. Many speech sounds contain an approximately steady-state region, where the formant patterns are not greatly influenced by the identities of the neighbouring sounds. Thus concatenation of vocoder representations of small units can be improved if each unit represents the transition from one phone to the next, rather than a single phone in isolation. Storing transition regions requires the number of units stored to be of the order of the square of the number of individual phonemes of the language, so might typically be about 1600. This number makes it possible to achieve an unlimited vocabulary. As the individual units are quite short the storage disadvantage is not too serious.

Transition units have variously been described as **diphones, dyads** or **demi-syllables**. The general principles of all three are similar, but there are differences in detail between techniques developed by different research groups. Demisyllables need to be slightly more numerous than diphones, because they may need to provide several consonant clusters. The use of demisyllables can be a great advantage for languages like English, where consonant clusters are common, because some consonant phonemes are acoustically quite different when they occur in clusters, compared with when they are in simple sequences of alternating consonants and vowels.

Even with diphone-like methods, one still gets significant variation at the centre of phones (i.e. at the diphone boundaries) according to the identities of the adjacent phonemes. The effect of this variation is that there would often be a considerable discontinuity in the acoustic specification where two diphones might join. Consider the words 'well', 'Ben', 'bell' and 'when'. The /w/ and /l/ phonemes are normally associated with quite long formant transitions, as a result of the large articulatory movements associated with these consonants. On the other hand the consonants /b/ and /n/ involve much more rapid transitions. In the middle of 'well', therefore, the normal articulatory position associated with the isolated form of the /e/ phoneme is

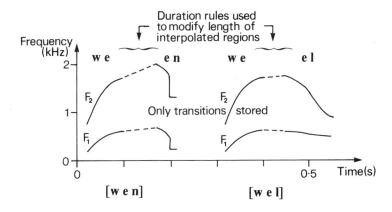

Fig. 5.2   Interpolation between formant coded diphones, to reduce discontinuity effects at junctions.

not reached, whereas in 'Ben' any undershoot will be quite minor. It is obvious, therefore, that a diphone for [we] appropriate for 'well' would not join correctly to the [en] diphone that was appropriate for 'when'. This difficulty can be eased by storing alternative forms of many of the diphones, but another approach is to store minimal length transitions and interpolate the synthesis parameters between the ends of the stored diphones, as illustrated in Fig. 5.2.

Current performance of complete text-to-speech systems using LPC-coded diphones and related methods is comparable with the better examples of the completely rule-based systems using formant synthesizers, which are described in the next chapter. Diphone methods have the advantage that the individual message parts are derived directly from human utterances, and therefore might be expected to be inherently natural-sounding. However, they also have some insuperable disadvantages. As these methods are vocoder-based, their underlying quality cannot be better than the vocoder method employed. If careful hand-editing is used to correct analysis errors it is possible to use a formant vocoder to generate the diphones, with its better modelling of speech acoustics. However, mainly because of the ease of analysis and availability of very low-cost synthesis chips, LPC diphones are the most widely used. The underlying quality is then limited to that possible from an LPC vocoder. The argument that naturally-derived transitions are inherently better is misleading, because there will be so many diphone junctions that do not fit together properly.

In human speech, durations of sounds vary considerably according to their positions in relation to the prosodic pattern of the sentence they are in. The transition durations are likely to vary less, because the inherent limitations in the speed of articulatory movements will prevent speeding up in proportion to speed of speaking. There is no doubt, however, that transitions produced at one rate of articulation will not be of exactly the same form as would be produced at a very different speed. Thus diphone methods may be less suitable for systems in which it is required to vary the speed of talking.

5.5 HARDWARE REQUIREMENTS

Stored coded waveform systems typically code the speech at 16 – 32 kbits/s. Assuming the lower figure, 1 Mbyte will store about 8 minutes of speech. This duration would be suitable for a reasonable range of pre-determined messages, and could be sufficient for an announcing system with a large variety of alternative words used in a few standard sentence types, such as for routine railway station announcements. For a larger set of messages, a disc drive might be preferable to semiconductor memory, provided disc access time can be kept short enough.

The decoders for use with simple waveform storage are extremely cheap and many are available as single-chip devices. The word selection and switching systems require no expensive components, so memory costs are likely to be dominant for a complete system.

For a system providing information to the general public through the telephone network the economics of system design are very different. In this case, many enquirers may be accessing the system simultaneously, all wanting different messages. Each access line will require its own switching circuits and a waveform decoder. However, the memory can be common to the whole system, and if the number of channels is very large the memory cost will contribute little to the cost per channel. For multi-channel systems it becomes practicable to provide a much wider range of messages using a waveform storage technique, but disc memory becomes more difficult to use because the total data rate and frequency of head movements would probably be too high.

LPC vocoder methods save roughly a factor of ten on memory size and memory data rate compared with waveform storage, and the requirement for the LPC synthesizer involves only one integrated circuit per output channel and adds little to the cost. If LPC coding is used with diphone synthesis for a complete text-to-speech system, the memory requirement for the diphones from one speaker of a single language is likely to be less than 100 Kbytes. The total hardware needed for the low-level synthesis part of the system would then be significantly less than would be used for the orthographic-to-phonetic conversion part, which is discussed in the next chapter.

SUMMARY
Chapter 5

Message synthesis from stored waveforms is a long-established technique for providing a limited range of information in the form of speech. The technical quality of the speech can be high, but it is not possible to produce good results for a wide range of message types by concatenating small units such as words.

Memory costs prevent waveform concatenation from being useful for large amounts of stored speech, but vocoder methods can reduce the memory by a factor of ten. Vocoders also give the possibility of varying pitch and timing, and joining words together more fluently.

Synthesis from vocoded diphones gives complete flexibility of message content, but is still limited by the inherent vocoder quality and by the difficulty of making the diphones represent all the different co-articulation effects that occur in different phonetic environments. Methods of producing a phonetic specification for the input to a diphone system are the same as for synthesis by rule.

The hardware cost for synthesis from stored human speech is dominated by the memory requirements except for multi-channel systems.

EXERCISES
Chapter 5

E5.1 Discuss the advantages and disadvantages of message synthesis by waveform concatenation.

E5.2 Why is it often beneficial to use vocoders in concatenation synthesis?

E5.3 What are the advantages and disadvantages of diphone synthesis and related techniques?

6

SPEECH SYNTHESIS BY RULE

6.1 INTRODUCTION

When human beings speak there are many factors that control how the acoustic output is related to the linguistic content of their utterances. At one level, there are the constraints determined by the physiology of their vocal apparatus. Although the physiology is generally similar between people, there are also clear differences of detail, partly related to age and sex, but also caused by various genetic differences between individuals.

For a given vocal system, the speech depends on the sequence of muscular actions that control the articulatory gestures. These gestures are learnt from early childhood, and their details are determined partly by the properties of the inherited central nervous system, but also very much by the speech environment in which the child grows up. The latter feature is entirely responsible for determining the inventory of available phonetic productions of any individual, which is closely tied to his/her native language.

At a higher level, the relationship between the ideas to be expressed with the choice of words, with their pitch, intensity and timing, is entirely determined by the language.

In acquiring competence in speech the human has two forms of feedback. On the one hand, auditory self-monitoring is paramount for comparing the acoustic patterns produced with those heard as model utterances. The second main form of feedback is the response by other human beings to imperfect utterances produced during language acquisition. Once the right types of utterances can be produced and the necessary gestures have been learnt, kinesthetic feedback can be used for detailed control of articulatory positions, and can ensure continuation of competent speech even if auditory feedback is not available for any reason.

All the above aspects of speech acquisition imply that the human develops a set of rules at many different levels, to convert concepts to speech. Although some parts of these rules are determined by inherited physiology and some by learning from the environment, it is not easy to separate these two aspects. However, it is clear that there must be a set of rules to guide humans generating speech, although in many cases the utterances will be modified by chance or by creative variation within the limits of what is acceptable to retain the desired effect on the listeners. To embody the complete process of human speaking, these rules must be fantastically complicated – particularly in the linguistic process of expressing subtle shades of meaning by choice of words and prosody. Although not trivial, sufficient rules for conversion of phoneme sequences to acoustic specifications are much easier to determine.

Speech synthesis by rule aims to imitate typical human rules well enough to produce synthetic speech that is acceptable to human listeners. The input can be at various levels, depending on the application. At the highest level, **synthesis from concept** requires a method of coding concepts in a machine and conversion through many stages to produce the speech. **Synthesis from text** should be able to apply the rules used by a good reader in interpreting written text and producing speech. In its most advanced form such a system should be able to apply semantic interpretation, so that the manner of speaking appropriate for the text can be conveyed where this is not immediately obvious from the short-span word sequences alone. At some stage either type of system will need a specification in phonemic units, with additional information about the required prosodic detail. For some applications this lower level can also provide a useful form of message input. When special effects are required, it can even be useful to specify input to synthesis rules at the level of the phonetic detail, but still to use rules to go from the phonetic specification to the speech waveform.

A characteristic of all systems considered in this chapter is that they do not store utterances of human speech in any form, although they do, of course, normally make extensive use of human utterances for guidance in formulating the rules.

6.2 ACOUSTIC–PHONETIC RULES

Human speech is produced as a result of muscular control of the articulators. The acoustic properties caused by even quite simple gestures can, however, be very complicated. For example, in the release of a stop consonant, such as [t], there can be very noticeable acoustic differences caused by slight variation of the relative timing of the tongue movement away from the alveolar ridge and the bringing together of the vocal folds in preparation for the voicing of a following vowel. If the **voice onset time** (VOT) is short there will be very little aspiration, and the perceptual quality will be much closer to [d]. Because the voicing then starts during the early stages of the tongue movement, it excites the transition of the first formant, which can be clearly seen on spectrograms. For a longer VOT the glottis will be wide open at release, and the resultant greater air flow gives rise to aspiration, i.e. turbulent noise excitation of the higher formants, for 60–100 ms.

The complex consequences of simple gestures have led people to suggest that rules for the phonetic level of synthesis would be much easier to specify in articulatory terms, for feeding an articulatory synthesizer. This viewpoint obviously has merit, but articulatory rules have not been generally adopted in practical speech synthesis systems for a number of reasons.

The most fundamental argument against using articulatory rules is that when humans acquire speech it is the auditory feedback that modifies their behaviour, without the speaker being consciously aware of the articulatory gestures. There are frequent cases of significantly non-standard articulatory strategies being used by some individuals to produce particular phonetic events. Although careful analysis sometimes reveals that the articulation of such people produces acoustic properties that differ consistently from the norm, the differences are not sufficient to cause phonetic confusion and will frequently not be noticed. In other cases the differences from the normal acoustic pattern are within the variation that occurs naturally between users of the more common articulation, and are not even detectable perceptually. The prime example of differing articulation for similar phonetic percepts occurs in the case of a good ventriloquist, who can produce a full range of speech sounds without externally obvious mouth movements. In developing an articulatory synthesis-by-rule system, it is thus not often easy to decide what the articulatory gestures should be for any particular phonetic event.

The second argument against using articulatory synthesis is merely the difficulty of accurate measurement of articulatory gestures. Various techniques are available, such as X-rays, electro-myography, fibre-scopes etc., but all are inconvenient to use and of limited accuracy. By contrast, synthesis methods that specify sounds directly in terms of measurable acoustic properties can have their control rules simply related to the acoustic features that are required, even though these features might be quite complicated in some cases. It is not then necessary even to consider the possible underlying articulatory gestures.

The third main reason for not using articulatory synthesis for machine voice output is that existing articulatory synthesizers have been much less successful than formant-based methods for modelling the perceptually important acoustic features (as already mentioned in Chapter 2).

6.2.1 Rules for formant synthesizers

For the reasons outlined above, most acoustic–phonetic rule systems are designed for directly driving some form of formant synthesizer. The input at this level is normally a sequence of allophones, each associated with prosodic information to specify duration, pitch and possibly also intensity. Allophonic variation in speech arises from two causes, both of which are normally systematic in operation. The first cause results from the phonological rules of a language, which may specify that a particular **extrinsic** allophone of a phoneme should be used in certain environments, even though other allophones could be produced by a speaker without much difficulty. The second cause, giving rise to **intrinsic** allophones, is a direct consequence of the constraints of articulation. The actual formant frequencies in a short vowel are greatly influenced by the articulatory gestures for the consonants on either side, and in consequence the acoustic properties in the centre of the sound representing a particular vowel phoneme may differ substantially for different consonant environments. The extrinsic allophones must obviously be specified by the input to a phonetic rule system, but it is normally possible to generate many of the co-articulation effects that give rise to intrinsic allophones automatically as a consequence of the way the rules operate.

Phonetic rule systems have been developed in a number of laboratories, and some are now incorporated in commercial text-to-speech products. In some cases the researchers have found it is advantageous to write a special notation for expressing the rules, to facilitate writing rule systems for a variety of languages. In others the rules have been written in a standard algorithmic computer language (such as Pascal or Fortran), with large numbers of conditional expressions to determine what synthesizer control signals should be generated for each type of phonetic event. A third approach is to have a very small number of computational procedures, driven by a large set of tables to represent the inventory of possible allophones. The numbers from the tables are then used by the computation to determine how all the synthesizer control signals should vary for any particular allophone sequence. An example of this table-driven method will be described in more detail, to illustrate the types of rules that are typically found useful.

6.2.2 Table-driven phonetic rules

The rules described in this section are appropriate for the type of parallel-formant synthesizer illustrated in Fig. 2.15. They are based on the technique described by Holmes, Mattingly and Shearme (1964) for a simpler parallel synthesizer. The following description includes some minor improvements to the computational algorithm given in the 1964 paper.

The synthesizer control parameters are calculated as a succession of frames, each of which has a duration of 10 ms. The input to the system comprises the sequence of speech sounds required, and for each sound there is a duration (in frames), and a specification of how to derive the fundamental frequency contour. There is also an option to vary the loudness of each sound from its default value.

This table-driven system is based on the idea that most speech sounds can be associated with some target acoustic specification, which might often not be reached, but which can be regarded as an ideal that would be aimed for in long isolated utterances. Simple vowels and continuant consonants are obvious examples where this concept seems appropriate. The target values for the ten synthesizer control signals specified for Fig. 2.15 are stored in the table for each such phone.

Other sounds, such as diphthongs and stop consonants, clearly have a sequence of acoustic properties, and each member of the sequence may be associated with a target specification and some transition rules for changing between targets. These sounds would be represented by a sequence of two or more component parts, each having its own table. Because a table in this system sometimes corresponds to a complete phone, and sometimes only to part of a phone, the term **phonetic element** has been used to describe the chunk of sound generated by the use of one table.

The table for each phonetic element also contains information relating to how transitions between target values are calculated around the boundaries between phonetic elements. In general, for transitions between a consonant and a vowel, it is the identity of the consonant that decides the nature of the transition. For example, nasal consonants have acoustic properties that change only slightly during the oral occlusion, but cause rapid changes at the boundary between consonant and vowel and fairly rapid but smooth formant transitions during the vowel. Fricative-vowel boundaries, on the other hand, can also have quite clearly discernible formant transitions during the frication. Types of transition are largely independent of what vowel is involved, although the actual numerical parameter values in each transition obviously depend on the associated vowel target value.

The Holmes-Mattingly-Shearme (HMS) system was designed to achieve the above properties without requiring special tables for each possible vowel/consonant combination. As the type of transition in a vowel–consonant (VC) or consonant–vowel (CV) sequence is determined mainly by the consonant, the table entries associated with the consonant are used to define the transition type. The only quantities used from the vowel tables are their target values. The operation of a transition calculation in the HMS system is explained below.

Consider a transition between a consonant, [w], and a vowel, [e], for the second-formant frequency parameter. Appropriate values for the targets of the two sounds might be 750 Hz and 2000 Hz, respectively. The system has a nominal boundary, where the two elements join, and has a method for calculating the parameter value at that boundary, taking into account the target value for the vowel and the identity of the consonant. The values either side of the boundary are derived by simple interpolation between the boundary value and the two target values, where the two interpolations are carried out over times that are specified in the consonant table. For each parameter the table for [w] will contain:

1 its own target value;
2 the proportion of the vowel target used in deriving the boundary value;

3 a 'fixed contribution' to the boundary value, specified for that consonant;

4 the transition duration within the consonant (in frames); and

5 the transition duration within the vowel (in frames).

The [w] table might have the following values for F_2: target=750 Hz, proportion=0.5, fixed contribution=350 Hz, internal duration=4, external duration=10. As F_2 for the [e] is 2000 Hz, the boundary value is 350+0.5×2000, which is 1350 Hz. The complete transition would then be as shown in Fig. 6.1. For simplicity, this diagram does not illustrate the level quantization or time quantization that will always be used in any practical system of this type. As specified by the algorithm, the transition calculation is of exactly the same form for CV and VC pairs. To a first approximation, this symmetry is reasonable as the articulatory movement between the vowel and consonant configurations are likely to be of broadly similar form irrespective of the direction of the change. However, where marked asymmetries are found in human speech they can be provided by splitting the consonant and using a pair of successive tables for consonants in VCV sequences.

Different values in the tables are used to achieve appropriate transitions for other control signals, and different tables are provided for all other vowels and consonants.

Of course, speech does not consist entirely of alternating consonants and vowels. Consonants often occur in clusters, and vowel sequences also occur, both within diphthongs and between syllables or words. The HMS system makes provision for these events by associating every phonetic element with a **rank**. Some phonemes which are undoubtedly consonants from a phonological point of view, such as [w], are acoustically more like vowels, and hence will contain formant transitions caused by adjacent consonants just

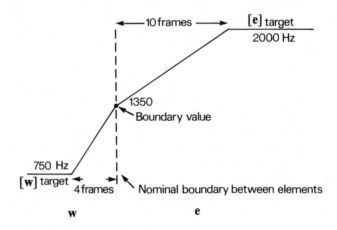

Fig. 6.1 Second-formant transition for the sequence [we], using the Holmes-Mattingly-Shearme (HMS) rule system.

as vowels will. Consonants such as stops will also tend to cause formant transitions in fricatives. The ranking system gives highest rank to those elements which have the strongest effect in determining the nature of transitions, and lowest rank to vowels. For any sequence of two elements the transition calculation is as described above; the table of the higher-rank element is used to determine the nature of the transition, and the table of the lower-rank element is used only to provide parameter targets. Where two consecutive elements have the same rank, the earlier one is arbitrarily regarded as dominant.

Overlapping transitions

The input to phonetic level synthesis is required to specify a duration for each element. It can happen that the transition durations as specified in the tables are so long in relation to the element duration that there is not time for the

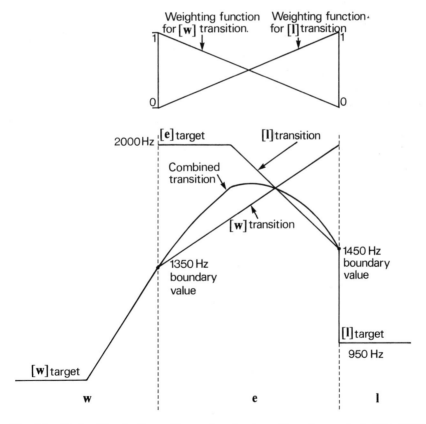

Fig. 6.2   Method for dealing with overlapping transitions in a variant of the HMS technique.

Element name = Q

	Tgt.	Prop.	F.C.	I.D.	E.D.
F_N	250	1	0	63	0
A_{LF}	1	1	-10	0	3
F_1	900	1	0	63	0
A_1	1	1	-10	0	3
F_2	2100	1	0	63	0
A_2	1	1	-10	0	3
F_3	2900	1	0	63	0
A_3	1	1	-10	0	3
A^{HF}	1	1	-10	0	3
V	1	1	0	63	0
Rank	63				

Element name = l

	Tgt.	Prop.	F.C.	I.D.	E.D.
F_N	250	0.5	125	0	6
A_{LF}	49	0	1	0	0
F_1	350	0.5	225	0	6
A_1	46	0	-2	0	0
F_2	950	0.5	450	0	6
A_2	47	0	12	0	0
F_3	2500	0.5	1250	0	6
A_3	50	0	15	0	0
A_{HF}	47	0	12	0	0
V	63	0	0	0	0
Rank	11				

Element name = w

	Tgt.	Prop.	F.C.	I.D.	E.D.
F_N	250	0.5	125	4	4
A_{LF}	51	0.5	23	4	4
F_1	200	0.5	50	4	6
A_1	43	0.5	22	4	4
F_2	750	0.5	350	4	10
A_2	40	0.5	20	4	4
F_3	2000	0.5	1000	4	4
A_3	36	0.5	18	4	4
A_{HF}	1	0.5	0	4	4
V	63	0	0	0	0
Rank	10				

Element name = z

	Tgt.	Prop.	F.C.	I.D.	E.D.
F_N	250	0.5	125	2	3
A_{LF}	36	0	1	0	0
F_1	275	0.5	150	2	3
A_1	33	0	-2	0	0
F_2	1700	0.5	950	2	3
A_2	37	0	12	0	0
F_3	2550	1	0	2	3
A_3	40	0	15	0	0
A_{HF}	57	0	12	0	0
V	32	1	-31	10	2
Rank	20				

Element name = e

	Tgt.	Prop.	F.C.	I.D.	E.D.
F_N	250	0.5	125	4	4
A_{LF}	52	0.5	27	4	4
F_1	650	0.5	325	4	4
A_1	49	0.5	26	4	4
F_2	2000	0.5	1000	4	4
A_2	48	0.5	24	4	4
F_3	2500	0.5	1250	4	4
A_3	53	0.5	27	4	4
A_{HF}	54	0.5	27	4	4
V	63	0	0	0	0
Rank	2				

Fig. 6.3 Table entries for five phonetic elements in a modified HMS system.

element to contain both the initial and final transitions without them overlapping in time. This effect is illustrated in Fig. 6.2 for the F_2 transition of the sequence [wel] (the word 'well'). The original HMS paper advocated a very crude method of producing some part of transition in such cases, but a more satisfactory method is as follows. For the element under consideration ([e] in Fig. 6.2), first construct separately that part of each transition which lies within the specified duration for the element, filling in the target value if necessary for the remainder of the frames of the element. Then construct the final parameter track by taking a weighted sum of the two component transitions over the duration of the element. The weighting function goes linearly from 1 to 0 for the initial transition, and from 0 to 1 for the final transition. The results of the linear weighting function applied to the linear transitions is to make the final components of the two transitions parabolic.

Examples of table entries for the 10 parameters for a few typical elements are shown in Fig. 6.3, and the resultant parameter tracks generated for the word 'wells' for F_1, A_1, F_2 and A_2 are shown in Fig. 6.4. The graphs in Fig. 6.4 include the time quantization into frames and the amplitude quantization of each parameter into 6-bit values. The phonemic significance of the element names shown in Figs 6.3 and 6.4 is obvious from the conventions of English orthography, except for Q which is used to signify silence.

The method of calculating parameter tracks in this table-driven system is extremely versatile. By suitable choice of table entries a very wide variety of transitions, appropriate for formant frequencies, formant amplitudes and

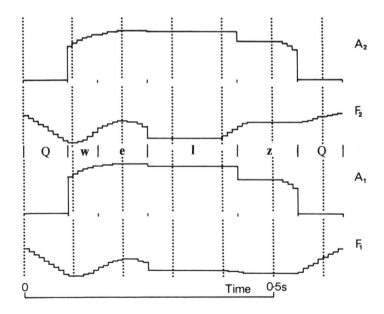

Fig. 6.4 Tracks of four parameters for the word 'wells', [welz], generated from the tables given in Fig. 6.3.

degree of voicing, can be constructed. The dominance system, determined by the ranks, is capable of providing many of the co-articulatory effects that occur, particularly where high-ranking consonants are adjacent to vowel-like sounds. However, it is obvious that values chosen to suit CV boundaries will not normally give sensible results if used to define the transitions between, for example, pairs of stop consonants, or between stops and nasals.

The system described above can be vastly improved by having different elements provided for different allophones of some of the phonemes. Element selection rules can then be used to take into account the phonetic environment of every phoneme in determining what element or sequence of elements should be used to specify the appropriate allophone. Without these selection rules around 60 elements are needed to provide one element or element sequence for each English phoneme. Increasing this number to around 200, where many of the extras are provided specifically to deal with the particular problems that would otherwise occur with consonant clusters, can provide a great improvement in quality. This increase only requires a modest amount of extra memory, and does not significantly increase the cost of a speech synthesis system, once the table values have been determined. The number of elements is far less than the number of items needed in a diphone system because so much of the co-articulation between vowels and consonants can be provided without specifying multiple allophones.

As it stands, the technique described above does not deal with co-articulation spreading across several phonemes. For example, lip-rounding for [w] is often maintained for several of the following speech sounds if none of them specifically requires spread lips. Here again, however, element selection rules can take into account remote phonetic environment to generate a suitable allophone in each case.

6.2.3 Optimizing phonetic rules

So far the usual method of choosing rules for the acoustic–phonetic part of a rule system has required the skill of an experimental phonetician assisted by instruments such as a spectrograph. Human subjective judgment provides, of course, the ultimate criterion of success, but it is very dangerous to rely too much on listening to guide small improvements because the listener easily gets perceptually saturated by repeated listening to the same short utterance. Phonetic theory, specifying the normal acoustic consequences of various articulatory events, has been widely used to formulate initial sets of rules for subsequent improvement. It can, however, be restrictive to structure a rule system primarily to deal with phonetic generalizations, because further study of imperfections of the rules may in many cases show the theory to be incorrect in detail, so requiring many special cases to be added to the rules.

Table-driven systems have a very large number of table values to be determined, and so at first sight it would seem that preparing rules for this method involves far more work than incorporating rules derived from theory directly in a computer program. However, it is quite practicable to use theory to guide the choice of initial table entries, and the experimenter can then introduce exceptions as they are shown to be necessary merely by modifying selected table entries.

Automatic adjustment of phonetic rules

Another possibility for adjusting phonetic rules is to prepare a fairly large corpus of phonetically transcribed speech data, and to analyse it in terms of the parameters that are calculated by the rules (e.g. formant frequencies and amplitudes). The same phonetic sequence can then be generated by the current set of rules, and the rules successively modified to achieve the optimal fit to the natural data, using an automatic process.

This method is potentially very powerful, but many problems have to be overcome before it can be applied for a practical rule system. One obvious problem, of aligning the time scales of the natural and synthesized parameters, can be solved by using the method of **dynamic programming** described in Chapter 7. Apart from the inconvenience of phonetically transcribing a large amount of speech, a major handicap to this technique is the difficulty of deciding in advance how many different allophones will be needed to achieve good rule synthesis for each phoneme. Until the allophonic variation has been decided, including the rules for selection of the allophones depending on phonemic environment, it will not be possible to transcribe the natural speech correctly. In due course it might also be possible to automate the choice of allophones, simply by allocating a new allophone for a particular phonemic environment whenever it is found that the rules match the natural data less well for one environment compared with others.

6.2.4   Rules for different speaker types

The process for deriving rules assumes that one has already decided on the type of talker one wishes to model. In a practical rule system the user may want many different types of voice for different occasions, and in particular may wish to switch from male to female or *vice versa*. Although the phonetic descriptions of male and female speech for the same accent are very similar, their acoustic realizations are quite different. The fundamental frequency of female speech is normally about an octave higher than for male speech. Because of a shorter vocal tract, the formant frequencies are also higher, usually by about 20%. The different dimensions of the vocal folds in a female larynx also cause the voiced excitation spectrum to be different in female speech, with far less power at the frequencies of the higher formants.

It seems almost certain that most of the effects mentioned above are systematic, so that transformations could be devised for converting rule systems between male and female speech. However, attempts so far to generate acceptable voice quality of female speech from male rules have had only limited success. It has been suggested by various workers that at least a part of the speech differences between the sexes is socially conditioned, in that the two sexes actually learn different styles of speech. If this effect is significant it could account for some of the difficulty in devising rule transformations between the sexes.

6.3 INTENSITY RULES

A large proportion of the intensity variations between phones depends merely on the identity of the phone being considered. For example, voiceless fricatives are fairly weak, and most vowels are quite strong. Those variations can easily be incorporated in the rules for generating the phones, and therefore do not require to be specified in the input to the acoustic–phonetic system. Intensity specifications could, however, be desirable as an optional modification to the default intensity for each allophone.

There are three obvious classes of intensity variation that may be desirable. First, for some applications it may be required to vary the overall loudness in a way that gives the impression of variation of vocal effort by the synthetic talker. This variation does not have the same effect as applying an overall scale change to the output waveform, because the spectral balance of the excitation changes with vocal effort. Loud speech has relatively more power in the higher-frequency region. The second factor affecting intensity is stress. Stressed syllables in a sentence are normally a little louder than unstressed syllables, although a part of this increase is simply a consequence of the increase of voiced excitation power that automatically arises from the pitch increase often associated with stressed syllables. The third cause of intensity change is the result of the lowering of vocal effort that normally occurs towards the end of each breath group.

In general, the above intensity variations involve changes of only a few dB from phone to phone, and most current synthesis-by-rule systems completely ignore them without serious damage to the output quality. However, the small intensity changes that might be desirable could easily be provided by rule if the syllable stress pattern and position in the breath group were known.

6.4 DURATION RULES

Acoustic–phonetic rules of the type described above require the duration associated with each phone to be supplied in the input specification.

However, the durations associated with phonemes vary according to a wide variety of different factors.

The inherent durations of different speech sounds differ considerably. Some vowels are intrinsically short and others long. The vowels in the words 'bit' and 'beet' in English differ in this way. Diphthongs are usually longer than monophthongs, and the various consonant sounds also show systematic differences.

Durations differ according to speed of speaking, but sounds which are mainly steady in character, such as fricatives and vowels, are likely to be more dependent on speed of speaking than intrinsically transient sounds, such as the bursts of stop consonants.

If a particular word in a sentence is emphasized, its most prominent syllable is normally lengthened.

Durations of phones vary according to their positions in a word, particularly if there are several syllables.

Words at the end of an utterance generally tend to be said more slowly than if they precede other words in the same utterance.

Vowels before voiced consonants are normally longer than occurrences of the same vowels before unvoiced consonants. For example, in the English words 'feed' and 'feet' the vowel is substantially longer in 'feed'. There are also other systematic durational modifications that depend on the identities of neighbouring phones.

In a 'stress-timed' language such as English, there is a tendency for unstressed syllables to be slightly shorter if there are several of them between any pair of stressed syllables.

In devising timing rules it is necessary to assume that the stressed syllables are marked, and that some decision has been made about speed of speaking. It is then possible to derive a suitable duration for each phone by having some instrinsic duration, and to modify it by various amounts according to each of the circumstances mentioned above. The amount of the modification could, in general, depend on the circumstances causing it and on the identity of the phone whose duration is being calculated.

Several rule systems of the above type have been developed for English, and have been reasonably successful in producing acceptable timing patterns. It is possible that more experiments with adapting the duration changes for each of the causes mentioned could produce further improvements. However, rules of this type are not sufficiently elaborate to produce the rhythm that humans seem to adopt naturally in sentences that may contain rhyming clauses, or other systematic variations related to meaning. A more elaborate linguistic analysis of a sentence would be necessary to produce such effects.

There is a school of thought that English and other stress-timed languages tend to have a constant time interval between syllables carrying primary stress, irrespective of how many other syllables lie between them (these intervals are known as **feet**). Some workers have tried implementing duration rules to produce this effect, but they seem to have been less successful at producing acceptable utterances than systems using the type of duration modification scheme described in the previous paragraphs.

Other languages will have many differences in detail for the duration rules, although many of the factors are probably universal across most languages.

6.5 FUNDAMENTAL FREQUENCY RULES

The fundamental frequency of voiced speech, which determines the perceived pitch, is widely used by all languages to convey information that supplements the sequence of phonemes. In some languages, such as Chinese, pitch changes are used to distinguish different meanings for syllables that are phonetically similar. In most western languages pitch does not help directly in identifying words, but provides additional information, such as which words in a sentence should be most prominent, whether a sentence is a question, statement or command, the mood of the speaker, etc. Even for these western languages, the type of intonation pattern that is used to achieve particular effects varies considerably from one language to another, and even between accents of the same language.

It is obvious that the rules for choosing a suitable intonation pattern must be developed to suit the required language. For the purposes of this book, examples of the necessary types of rule will be given for English as spoken in south-east England.

Most sentences in English show a general tendency for pitch to fall gradually from beginning to end of each sentence, with many local variations around this trend. The most significant variations occur on words that the user wishes to be more prominent. In the case of polysyllabic words, there is normally one syllable that is given **primary stress**, and in consequence carries the main pitch movement. Other syllables of the word are either unstressed, or carry a less prominent **secondary stress**.

The normal structure of English is such that the last syllable carrying primary stress in any breath group is given the biggest pitch change, and is known as the **nuclear syllable**. Usually the **nuclear tone** (i.e. pitch pattern on the nuclear syllable) on a simple statement is a pitch fall, but a number of other patterns are possible to indicate other types of utterance. (The number of possible nuclear tones is at least three, but some workers have claimed that there are several more significantly different patterns.) The nuclear tone for a question expecting a yes/no answer shows a substantial pitch rise. On the non-final stressed syllables the pitch usually shows a local small rise and then continues its steady fall. The amount of this rise and the subsequent rate of fall can depend on the syntactic function of the word in the sentence: verbs, for example, generally have less pitch variation than nouns and adjectives. At the beginning of an utterance the pitch often starts fairly low, and then rises to a high value on the first stressed syllable.

In addition to these pitch changes caused by the pattern of stressed syllables, there are also smaller pitch variations that are influenced by the phonetic detail of an utterance. When voicing recommences after any voiceless consonant there is a tendency for the pitch to be a little higher for a few tens of milliseconds than it would be after a voiced consonant. Also, because of muscular interactions between the articulators and the larynx, some vowels tend to be of intrinsically higher pitch than others.

It is not too difficult to define rules for generating typical English nuclear tones, provided it is known which of the few alternative patterns is required in each breath group. These patterns can then be superimposed on the falling trend, with local variations of the type described above for the other stressed syllables and for the various phonetic effects. Although some research groups have demonstrated some very natural-sounding utterances with rule intonation generated in this way, to achieve these results the input to the intonation rule system has needed a very detailed specification of the utterance structure.

Intonation rules used in practical text-to-speech systems, although usually producing plausible pitch patterns, do not generally produce such natural-sounding speech, and the intonation usually sounds less 'interesting' than one would expect from a human talker. Much further research is needed to achieve really natural intonation for generation of speech from text, but it seems likely that a major limitation is the difficulty of making a sufficiently accurate linguistic analysis of the text to be able to provide the appropriate specification as input to the rules.

Speech synthesis from concept potentially overcomes this difficulty, because in the process of converting the concept into words one implicitly has a very detailed knowledge of the syntactic and semantic function of each word. However, synthesis from concept has so far received so little attention that it is too early to say whether these predictions will be borne out of practice.

6.6 TEXT ANALYSIS RULES

In a language such as English the relationship between the spellings of words and their phonemic transcription is extremely complicated. However, it is obvious that human readers must have some rules for relating spelling to phoneme sequences, because they can usually make a reasonable guess at the pronunciation of an unfamiliar word, which, if not completely right, will have the correct choice for most of the phonemes.

It is also clear that any general rules there are have many idiosyncratic exceptions, as exemplified by the different vowels in the words 'bead' and 'dead', and the fact that both of these vowels are valid for 'lead' to give two distinct meanings. There are also examples of a particular spelling of a two-syllable word, such as 'permit', having its primary stress on a different syllable, depending on whether it is being used as a noun or a verb. In this last example the phoneme sequence is the same in both cases.

Analysis of text for subsequent speech synthesis thus needs to decide on the appropriate phoneme sequence, and also decide on the allocation of stressed syllables within each word. If natural prosody is to be achieved it will also be necessary to determine the syntactic structure of each sentence, and in some cases even semantic analysis is also desirable.

6.6.1 Grapheme-to-phoneme conversion

The phonemic transcriptions of words which are obviously pronounced in a way that would not be predicted by any general rules need to be in a dictionary of exceptions. Many very common words of English are in this category, such as 'one', 'two', 'said', etc. However, it is not possible to put all conceivable valid words in a dictionary, even if the necessary large amount of computer memory were available, because new words are continually being created, many words in text are proper names that could not have been anticipated, and foreign words are often encountered. It is therefore necessary in any text-to-speech system to have a spelling-to-sound rule system for dealing with non-dictionary items. It cannot be guaranteed that these rules will always give the pronunciation that most people would regard as correct, but in the case of an unfamiliar word, a human reader will also often make errors. Usually these words are sufficiently rare and the nature of the error is such that the incorrect phoneme sequence is sufficient to indicate the intended word.

In English there are about 100 – 200 common words, such as articles, conjunctions, prepositions and auxiliary verbs, that serve to indicate the relationships between the words that carry the main information content of an utterance. These common words are often known as **function words**, and the others are referred to as **content words**. As function words do not normally carry any stress but content words do, it is necessary to include all function words in the dictionary and to label their entries appropriately. The default for words dealt with by spelling-to-sound rules can then be to allocate at least one stressed syllable.

As explained in section 6.5, a more natural intonation pattern is possible if the syntactic structure of a sentence is known, and so it could be advantageous to have most words in the dictionary, and to include an entry for the possible syntactic class of each word. However, a high proportion of English words can be used as both nouns and verbs, and many can also be adjectives, so very little definite information about syntax can be resolved without taking the relationships between content words and their associated function words into account. Although techniques of language processing are becoming available to make analyses of this type, they are still too complicated to be routinely applied in present-day speech output systems. For this reason designers of text-to-speech systems are not yet able to make use of much more than the distinction between content and function words in determining the prosody of utterances.

A high proportion of words in English can be combined with prefixes and/or suffixes to make other words, for which the pronunciations of the words with their affixes are closely related to the pronunciations of the root words. It therefore makes the dictionary much more powerful in determining the pronunciation of irregular words if it can be searched after the removal of any affixes. The pronunciation of any derived word can then be determined by the pronunciation of the root and the normal pronunciations of the affixes. For example, inclusion of the word 'prove' would enable the correct pronunciation of 'improvement', 'proving', etc. to be determined. (Note that it is necessary to take account of the fact that many words remove a final 'e' before the addition of some suffixes.)

A typical strategy for determining pronunciation is then as follows:

1 Test to see if the word is in the dictionary; if so, take the dictionary pronunciation and go to step **5**.
2 See if a standard affix can be removed.
3 If an affix was removed, return to step **1**.
4 When no more affixes are found, see if the root is in the dictionary; if so, take the dictionary pronunciation for the root, otherwise apply spelling-to-sound rules.
5 Add the pronunciations of any affixes that have been removed, taking into account any modification rules associated with the affixes (e.g. the suffix 'ion' changes the phonemic interpretation of the final /t/ sound of words like 'create').

At MIT during the 1970s a system called MITalk was developed (Allen, 1987) that took word decomposition much further than the affix stripping described above. In MITalk words are decomposed into **morphs**, which are the sub-parts of words that can be regarded as having some independent function of meaning. In many words, such as 'carrot', the whole word consists of a single morph. Others, such as 'lighthouse', have two or more. The addition of common affixes can vastly increase the number of morphs in a word, and 'antidisestablishmentarianism' has six if 'establish' is regarded as a single root morph.

The advantage of the morph decomposition method is that it can deal effectively with the many compound words of English, and cover a very high proportion of the total vocabulary while still keeping the dictionary of manageable size. Even so, many thousands of morphs are necessary to cover most written English, and even then many proper names, technical terms, etc. will be excluded. Many of the dictionary entries will, in fact, need to specify sequences of morphs, to deal with cases where the pronunciation of a sequence cannot be simply predicted from the pronunciations associated with the individual morphs.

6.6.2 Stress assignment

For many polysyllabic words of English the placement of primary and secondary stresses on the syllables can be determined using very complicated rules that depend on how many vowels there are in the word, how many consonants follow each vowel, the vowel lengths, etc. There are however, many words for which the normal rules do not apply, which is exemplified by the fact that some pairs of words are of similar structure yet are stressed differently. Examples are 'Canada' and 'camera', contrasting with 'Granada' and 'banana'.

The difficulty of getting reliable stress assignment is another reason for putting words in the dictionary, so that their stress markings can be pre-defined. The MITalk morph dictionary also carries stress marks, but the rules for working out the pronunciations of complete words have to take into account the fact that the stress pattern is often changed by combining morphs. For example, the addition of the suffix 'ity' to 'electric' moves the primary stress from the second syllable to the third.

Words such as 'permit', for which the stress assignment depends on syntax, ideally require the sentence to be correctly parsed. It seems likely that some form of syntactic tagging of surrounding words might be sufficient to determine the noun/verb choice in a fair proportion of cases, but many practical text-to speech systems do not yet include this facility.

6.7 PRE-PROCESSING OF NUMERALS, ABBREVIATIONS, ETC.

In a text-to-speech system for general application there will often be occurrences of numerals, abbreviations, and special symbols such as %, *, etc. It is therefore necessary to pass the text through a pre-processing stage that converts all such occurrences to pronounceable words, unless in particular cases it is better to remove them instead.

Rules for abbreviations can be quite straightforward if the abbreviations are known in advance and are in the dictionary. If not, the presence of full stops between the letters or the use of capitals can be taken as an indication that letter names should be pronounced separately. However, the latter criterion will not give the right result for headings in which ordinary words are spelt in capitals. One should possibly use the criterion that a single word in capitals surrounded by lower case words is an abbreviation, but a sequence of words in capitals is a heading. It is also reasonable to assume that a group of letters that does not conform to the normal permitted letter sequences in English words must be an abbreviation. Even when using all of these rules there might still be errors, such as if a pronounceable sequence like 'MIT' occurs in a capitalized heading and has not been included in the dictionary.

For numerals, there are many special cases depending on context. In many contexts 4-digit numbers beginning in 1 will be pronounced according to the conventions for dates, but in other cases will be 'one thousand' followed by the hundreds, tens and units. Telephone numbers in English are usually pronounced as a sequence of separate digits. A number with two decimal places will be pronounced as a sum of money if preceded by a pound or dollar symbol, but will otherwise include the word 'point'.

The best procedure for abbreviations and numerals, and the treatment of special symbols, will depend on the type of text that is fed into the system. To achieve good results the designer must either prepare the system for a particular restricted range of applications, or alternatively include a sufficiently elaborate analysis of the type of text so that the appropriate rules can be used in each case. Current text processing has not yet reached the stage where the latter approach is a practical option.

6.8 HARDWARE IMPLEMENTATION

Systems for synthesis from text involve a very large number of very complicated rules, and normally also require a very large pronouncing dictionary. Even so, in most cases the necessary program code and the storage of all the rules is unlikely to need more than about 50 Kbytes. The dictionary is unlikely to need an average of more than 30 bytes per word, so a complete system with a 10000 word dictionary might need 350 Kbytes of memory, most of which would not need very fast access.

The computation required is of three distinct types. At the output end, a formant synthesizer would these days normally be implemented using digital signal processing techniques. If the expected production volume justified the development cost, it would use a custom integrated circuit, but for smaller volumes would use a standard digital signal processor (DSP) device. In the former case only one chip would be needed, and in the latter the DSP would possibly need supplementing by a small number of support chips for memory and analogue output. Although the amount of arithmetic for the signal processing would be large, the calculations would be very repetitive and the hardware would be quite simple.

The acoustic–phonetic processing might require calculation of about 1000 parameter values per second, but would use fairly complicated rules. The speed of electronic circuits is such that these calculations would require only a fraction of the power of one standard 8-bit microprocessor.

All the higher levels require much more complicated rules, but the input and output data rates are very low (only about 20 symbols per second for each stage of the processing). Semantic processing is still insufficiently developed for it to be possible to predict the computational load needed, but if semantics are excluded there is sufficient time available in a simple processor to implement any likely high-level rules serially in real time.

For the above reasons the best of present-day capabilities for text to speech can be implemented easily on a single circuit board of moderate size. With special development of custom circuits and hybrid technology, such a device could be reduced to a PCB-mounted module only a few centimetres long.

6.9 CURRENT SYNTHESIS-BY-RULE CAPABILITIES

There are now many text-to-speech systems working in research laboratories, and also several commercial products. All of these systems have to use rules for converting the text to phonemic form, and many also use rules for the phonetic synthesis.

Current performance of the more complicated systems produces speech which is highly intelligible on material that has a simple linguistic content, but the phonetic detail is not as clear as one would like, the intonation rarely matches the naturalness of a human speaker, and the general quality seems 'machine-like'. On difficult material, or in the presence of background noise, the intelligibility falls far short of that from a good human reader of the same text.

It seems reasonable to assume, provided a good enough formant synthesizer is available, that detailed rule optimization will make the phonetic features almost perfect within a few years. The prosodic and pronunciation aspects are likely to be limited by the difficulties of analysing the semantics of the text for many years to come.

SUMMARY
Chapter 6

Human beings have acquired rules to convert from ideas to speech, and also to read from written text.

Machine rules for the same processes involve several levels.

The speech waveform generation is best done using a formant synthesizer. Rules can then convert from a detailed phonetic specification to control signals for the synthesizer. A convenient implementation is to store these rules as tables of numbers for use by a simple computational procedure.

Rules can be adapted for different speaker types, but so far with limited success.

Rules at the next level specify the duration and fundamental frequency pattern of each allophone, from information about the stressed syllables and sentence structure.

Above this level, the input can be text or concept, but most systems currently only deal with text input.

For English it is difficult to determine the correct pronunciation and stress pattern from ordinary text, but a pronouncing dictionary, possibly with morph decomposition, makes the task easier.

Because most of the more complicated rules only need to operate slowly, it is possible to implement a complete text-to-speech system on very low-cost hardware.

Current products give reasonably intelligible but somewhat unnatural speech, but significant improvements are expected soon.

EXERCISES
Chapter 6

E6.1 Discuss the benefits and difficulties that arise from using articulatory rules for speech synthesis.

E6.2 In view of the very large number of table entries that must be provided, why are table-driven phonetic rules practically convenient?

E6.3 How can allophonic variation be provided for in acoustic/phonetic synthesis rules?

E6.4 Explain the concept of 'rank' in the Holmes-Mattingly-Shearme synthesis technique.

E6.5 Discuss the relative importance of pitch, intensity and duration in prosodic rule systems.

E6.6 Describe a technique for converting from conventional to phonetic spelling for a language such as English, highlighting any special difficulties.

E6.7 Why should conventional orthography not be used as an intermediate representation in systems for synthesis from concept?

E6.8 Discuss the main influences on hardware cost in text-to-speech systems for English.

7

SPEECH RECOGNITION BY PATTERN MATCHING OF WHOLE WORDS

7.1 GENERAL PRINCIPLES

When a person utters a word, as we saw in Chapter 1, the word can be considered as a sequence of phonemes (the linguistic units) and the phonemes will be realized as phones. Because of inevitable co-articulation, the acoustic patterns corresponding to individual phones overlap in time, and therefore depend on the identities of their neighbours. Even for a word in isolation, therefore, the acoustic pattern is related in a very complicated way to the word's linguistic structure.

However, if the same person repeats the same isolated word on separate occasions, the pattern is likely to be generally similar, because the same phonetic relationships will apply. Of course, there will probably also be differences, arising from many causes. For example, the second occurrence might be spoken faster or more slowly; there may be differences in vocal effort; the pitch and its variation during the word could be different; one example may be spoken more precisely than the other, etc. It is obvious that the waveform of separate utterances of the same word may be very different. Spectrograms are likely to be less obviously different, because they better illustrate the resonances, which are closely related to the positions of the articulators. But even spectrograms will differ in detail as a result of all the above types of difference, and time-scale differences will be particularly obvious.

A well established approach to automatic speech recognition (ASR) is to store in the machine example acoustic patterns (called **templates**) for all the words to be recognized, usually spoken by the person who will subsequently use the machine. Any incoming word is compared in turn with all words in the store, and the one that is most similar is assumed to be the correct one. In general none of the templates will match perfectly, so to be successful this technique must rely on the incoming word being more similar to the correct template than to any of the possible alternatives.

It is obvious that in some sense the sound pattern of the correct word is likely to be a better match than a wrong word, because it is made by more similar articulatory movements. Exploiting this similarity is, however, critically dependent on how the word patterns are compared, i.e. on how the 'distance' between two word examples is calculated. For example, it would be useless to compare waveforms, because even very similar repetitions of a word will differ appreciably in waveform detail from moment to moment, largely as a result of the difficulty of repeating the intonation and timing exactly.

It is implicit in the above comments that it must also be possible to identify the start and end points of words that are to be compared.

7.2 DISTANCE METRICS

In this section we will consider the problem of comparing the templates with the incoming speech when we know that corresponding points in time will correspond to similar articulatory events. In effect, we appear to be assuming that the words to be compared are spoken in isolation at exactly the same speed, and that their start and end points can be reliably determined. In practice these assumptions will very rarely be justified, and methods of dealing with the resultant problems will be discussed later in the chapter.

In calculating a distance between two words it is usual to derive a short-term distance that is local to corresponding parts of the words, and to integrate this distance over the entire word duration. Parameters representing the acoustic signal must be determined over some span of time, during which the properties are assumed not to change much. In one such span of time the measurements can be represented as an ordered set of numbers, or **feature vector**, which can be regarded as representing a point in multi-dimensional space. The properties of a whole word can then be described as a succession of feature vectors (sometimes known as **frames**), each of which represents a time slice of, say 10 – 20 ms. The integral of the distance between the patterns then reduces to the sum of distances between corresponding pairs of feature vectors. To be useful, the distance must not be sensitive to small differences in intensity between otherwise similar words, and it should not give too much weight to differences in pitch. Those features of the acoustic signal that are determined by the phonetic properties should obviously be given more weight in the distance calculation.

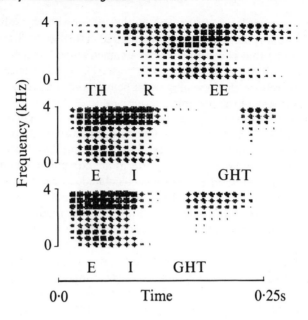

Fig. 7.1 Spectrogram displays of a 9-channel filter-bank analysis of one example of the word 'three' and two examples of 'eight'. It can be seen that the two eights are generally similar, except that the lower one has a much shorter gap for the [t] and a longer burst.

7.2.1 Filter-bank analysis

The most obvious approach in choosing a distance metric which has some of the desirable properties is to use some representation of the short-term power spectrum. It has been explained in Chapter 2 how the short-term spectrum can represent the effects of moving formants, excitation spectrum, etc.

Although in tone languages pitch needs to be taken into account, in western languages there is normally only slight correlation between pitch variations and the phonetic content of a word. The likely idiosyncratic variations of pitch that will occur from occasion to occasion means that except for tone languages it is normally safer to ignore pitch in the pattern-matching process. And even for tone languages it is probably desirable to analyse pitch variations separately from the effects of articulation. It is best, therefore, to make the bandwidth of the spectral resolution such that it will not resolve the harmonics of the fundamental of voiced speech. Because the excitation periodicity is evident in the amplitude variations of the output from a broad-band analysis, it is also necessary to apply some time smoothing to remove it. Such smoothing will also remove most of the fluctuations that result from randomness in turbulent excitation.

At higher frequencies the precise formant positions become less significant, and the resolving power of the ear (**critical bands**, see Chapter 3) is such that detailed spectral information is not available to human listeners at these frequencies. It is therefore permissible to make the spectral analysis less selective, such that the effective filter bandwidth is several times the typical harmonic spacing. The desired analysis can thus be provided by a set of band-pass filters whose bandwidths and spacings are roughly equal to critical bands and whose range of centre frequencies covers the frequencies most important for speech perception (say 300 – 5000 Hz). The total number of band-pass filters is therefore not likely to be more than about 20, and successful results have often been achieved with less.

The usual name for this type of speech analysis is **filter-bank** analysis. Whether it is provided by a bank of discrete filters, implemented in analogue or digital form, or is implemented by sampling the outputs from short-term Fourier transforms, is a matter of engineering convenience. Fig. 7.1 displays word patterns from a typical filter-bank analyser for two examples of one word and one example of another.

A consequence of removing the effect of the fundamental frequency and of using filters as wide as critical bands is to reduce the amount of information needed to describe a word pattern to much less than is needed for the waveform. Thus the computation in the pattern-matching process is much reduced.

7.2.2 Level normalization

Mean speech level normally varies by a few decibels over periods of a few seconds, and changes in spacing between the microphone and the speaker's mouth can also produce changes of several decibels. As these changes will be of no phonetic significance, it is desirable to minimize their effects on the distance metric. Use of filter-bank power directly gives most weight to more intense regions of the spectrum, where a 2 or 3 dB change will represent a very large absolute difference. On the other hand, a 3 dB difference in one of the weaker formants might be of similar phonetic significance, but will cause a very small effect on the power. This difficulty can be avoided to a large extent by representing the power logarithmically, so that similar power ratios have the same effect on the distance calculation whether they occur on intense or weak spectral regions. Most of the phonetically unimportant variations discussed above will then have much less weight in the distance calculation than the differences in spectrum level that result from formant movements etc.

Although comparing levels logarithmically is advantageous, care must be exercised in very low-level sounds, such as weak fricatives or during stop-consonant closures. At these times the logarithm of the level in a channel will depend more on the ambient background noise level than on the speech signal. If the speaker is in a very quiet environment the logarithmic level may suffer quite wide irrelevant variations as a result of breath noise or the rustle of clothing. A way of avoiding this difficulty is to add a small constant to the measured level before taking logarithms. The value of the constant would be chosen to dominate the greatest expected background noise level, but to be small compared with the level usually found during speech.

Differences in vocal effort will mainly have the effect of adding a constant to all components of the log spectrum, rather than changing the shape of the spectrum cross-section. Such differences can be made to have no effect on the distance metric by subtracting the mean of the logarithm of the spectrum level of each frame from all the separate spectrum components of the frame. In practice this amount of level compensation is undesirable because extreme level variations are of some phonetic significance. For example, a substantial part of the acoustic difference between [f] and any vowel is the difference in level, which could be as much as 30 dB. Recognition accuracy might well suffer if level differences of this magnitude were ignored. A useful compromise is to compensate only partly for level variations, by subtracting some fraction (say in the range 0.7 – 0.9) of the mean logarithmic level from each spectral channel. There are also several other techniques for achieving the same effect.

A suitable distance metric for use with a filter bank might be the sum of the squared differences between the logarithms of power levels in corresponding channels (i.e. the square of the **Euclidean distance** in the multi-dimensional space). To avoid the computational load of the squaring operations it is quite common merely to use the sum of the magnitudes of the differences in channel levels (sometimes known as the **city-block** metric because of its relationship to the distance in two dimensions between points in a rectangular street layout). This change to the metric reduces the relative weight given to large differences in single channels compared with smaller differences in many channels. Such performance comparisons as have been made have not shown any conclusive preference between the Euclidean and city-block metrics, but the squared Euclidean distance has certain theoretical attractions that will become clear in the next chapter. A graphical representation of the Euclidean distance between frames for the words used in Fig. 7.1 is shown in Fig. 7.2.

7.2.3 Other simple spectrally-based distance metrics

Because of the profound importance of the short-term spectrum in representing the acoustic consequences of phonetic events, it is almost essential that the acoustic analysis and distance metric should be related to spectral difference. But the simple filter bank, although fairly effective and very widely used, is only one of a range of possibilities. Even with a filter bank, it is possible to save computation by reducing the number of filters, or

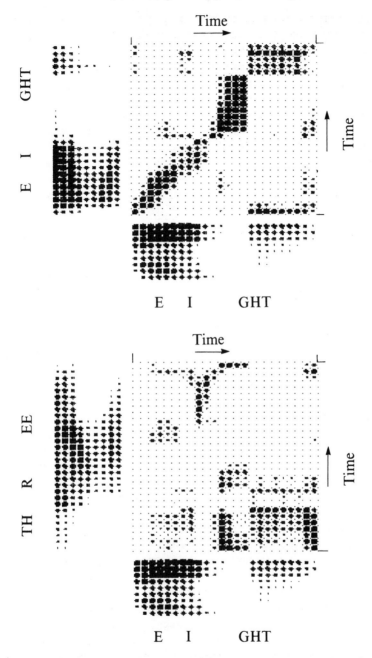

Fig. 7.2 Graphical representation of Euclidean distance between frames of the spectrograms shown in Fig. 7.1. The larger the blob the smaller the distance. It can be seen that there is a path of fairly small distances between the bottom left and top right when two examples of 'eight' are compared, but not when 'eight' is compared with 'three'.

quantizing their levels more coarsely. In general such changes are likely to degrade recognition performance to some extent, but may still be beneficial overall because of the resultant cost reduction. As an extreme example of simplification, it is possible to retain some indication of the spectral balance between high and low frequencies in the speech merely by measuring the zero-crossing rate of the waveform over a frame period. In this case the feature vectors would contain only two components – zero-crossing rate and some representation of intensity, but even such a crude system can be used to discriminate between a very small vocabulary of dissimilar words.

Another possible spectrum-derived analysis is an orthogonal transformation of the spectrum cross-section, as represented by the logarithmic channel levels, A_1 to A_n. A suitable transform is a discrete cosine transform, for reasons explained below:

$$C_0 = \sqrt{\frac{1}{n} \sum_{i=1}^{n} A_i}$$

$$C_j = \sqrt{\frac{2}{n} \sum_{i=1}^{n} A_i \cos\left(\frac{\pi j (i - 0.5)}{n}\right)} \tag{7.1}$$

for $j = 1$ to $n-1$.

For typical speech signals it is found that, in contrast with the original channel signals, the variation of the separate coefficients, C_j, tends to be uncorrelated, and most of the variance of the original channel data is carried by only the lowest three or four C_j coefficients. The C_0 term is proportional to the mean of the log channel signals, and thus represents the mean-level term discussed in section 7.2.2. Although the cosine transformation given by eqn (7.1) ensures that the Euclidean distance in transformed space is exactly equal to the distance between the sets of untransformed channel signals, the concentration of the variance in the lower-order terms means that higher-order terms are small and the distance is almost unaltered if they are ignored. Most of the small contribution from the higher-order terms will, in any case, probably be caused by phonetically irrelevant detail. The advantage in using a cosine or similar transform is thus that the higher-order transformed feature components can be ignored when calculating the distance, so simplifying the pattern-matching process. The disadvantage arises mainly in the presence of background noise. Because the transformation mixes signals from the low-level channels (caused by noise) with high-level channels (carrying the speech formants), there is no possibility of applying subsequent non-linear processing in the distance calculation to compensate for the lower reliability of the low-level signals. This aspect is discussed further at the end of this chapter.

7.2.4 Linear prediction analysis

An alternative commonly used analysis method related to the short-term spectrum is to derive linear prediction coefficients (usually called LPC analysis because of its origin in linear predictive coding, see Chapter 4). Although one possibility with LPC is to use the Euclidean distance between vectors of, for example, reflection coefficients, the process of inverse filtering inherent in LPC analysis gives another possible measure. If the short-term spectra of the two speech signals being compared are similar, it follows that inverse filtering of one signal with the prediction filter derived from the other will give a small residual. A quantity derived from the power in this residual, known as the **Itakura distance metric** (Itakura, 1975) can therefore be used as a measure of spectral similarity. The main advantage of the Itakura metric is the computational ease of linear prediction analysis. Many recognizers have been built using it, and they seem to give performance comparable with that obtained from recognizers using filter-bank methods. However, because there is less freedom to apply non-linear processing to combat noise, and because of the inherently uniform weighting LPC gives to low- and high-frequency features, it lacks the potential for elaboration that is available with a filter-bank front end.

7.2.5 Analysis based on models of auditory perception

As a general policy for automatic speech recognition, it seems desirable not to use features of the acoustic signal that are not used by human listeners, even if they seem to be reliably present in human productions, because they may be distorted by the acoustic environment or electrical transmission path without apparently causing the speech quality to be impaired. It is now well established that the frequencies of the speech formants, particularly the first and second, are vitally important phonetically. Their relative amplitudes are much less important, and the detailed structure of the lower-level spectral regions between formants is of almost no consequence. There would therefore seem to be potential for better performance in speech recognition if these factors could be taken into account in designing a distance metric. There is much current research in this general direction, and preliminary results suggest that these methods will offer substantial advantages. The more elaborate schemes take into account what is known about the lower levels of human auditory processing (see Chapter 3) to design acoustic analysis methods and distance metrics that give most weight to features known to be significant in human perception. The detail of these more elaborate methods of speech analysis is beyond the scope of this book, but they are dealt with in recent research literature. (See Chapter 11.)

7.3 END-POINT DETECTION FOR ISOLATED WORDS

The pattern comparison methods described above assume that the beginning and end points of words can be defined. In the case of words spoken in isolation in a quiet environment it is possible to use some simple level threshold to determine start and end points. There are, however, problems with this approach when words start or end with a very weak sound, such as [f]. In such cases the distinction in level between the background noise and the start or end of the word may be slight, and so the end points will be very unreliably defined. Even when a word begins and ends in a strong vowel, it is common for speakers to precede the word with slight noises caused by opening the lips, and to follow the word by quite noisy exhalation. If these spurious noises are to be excluded the level threshold will certainly have to be set high enough also to exclude weak unvoiced fricatives. Some improvement in separation of speech from background noise can be obtained if the spectral properties of the noise are also taken into account. However, there is no reliable way of determining whether low-level sounds that might immediately precede or follow a word should be regarded as an essential part of that word without simultaneously determining the identity of the word.

Of course, even when a successful level threshold criterion has been found, it is necessary to take into account that some words can have a period of silence within them. Any words (such as 'containing' and 'stop') containing unvoiced stop consonants at some point other than the beginning belong to this category. The level threshold can still be used in such cases, provided the end-of-word decision is delayed by the length of the longest possible stop gap, to make sure the word has really finished. When isolated words with a final unvoiced stop are used for pattern matching, a more serious problem, particularly for English, is that the stop consonant burst is sometimes, but not always, omitted by the speaker. Even when the end points are correctly determined, the patterns being compared for words which are nominally the same will then often be inherently different.

Although approximate end points can be determined for most words, it is apparent from the above comments that they are often not reliable.

7.4 ALLOWING FOR TIME-SCALE VARIATIONS

Up to now we have assumed that words to be compared will be of the same length, and corresponding times in separate utterances of a word will represent the same phonetic features. In practice speakers vary their speed of speaking, and often do so non-uniformly so that equivalent words of the same total length may differ in the middle. This time-scale uncertainty is made worse by the unreliability of end-point detection. It would not be unusual for two patterns of apparently very different length to have the underlying speech

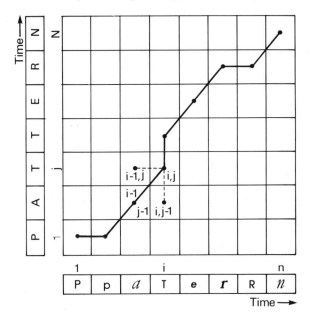

Fig. 7.3 Illustration of a time-alignment path between two words that differ in time scale. Any point *i,j* can have three predecessors as shown.

at the same speed and merely to have a final fricative cut short in one case as a result of a slight difference of level.

Some early implementations of isolated word recognizers tried to compensate for the time-scale variation by a uniform time normalization to ensure that all patterns being matched were of the same length. This process is a great improvement over methods such as truncating the longer pattern when it is being compared with a shorter one, but the performance of such machines was undoubtedly limited by differences in time scale. More recently a technique has been developed which is capable of matching one word on to another in a way which applies the optimum non-linear time-scale distortion to achieve the best match at all points. The mathematical technique used is known as **dynamic programming** (DP), and when applied to speech recognition the process is often referred to as **dynamic time warping** (DTW).

7.5 DYNAMIC PROGRAMMING FOR TIME ALIGNMENT

Assume that an incoming speech pattern and a template pattern are to be compared, having n and N frames respectively. Some distance metric can be used to calculate the distance $d(i,j)$, between frame i of the incoming speech and frame j of the template. To illustrate the principle, in Fig. 7.3 the two sets of feature vectors of the words have been represented by letters of the word 'pattern'. Differences in time scale have been represented by repeating or omitting letters of the word, and the fact that feature vectors will not be identical, even for corresponding points of equivalent words, is represented by using different type styles for the letters. It is, of course assumed in this explanation that all styles of the letter 'a' will yield a lower value of distance between them than, say, the distance between an 'a' and any example of a letter 'p'. To find the total difference between the two patterns one requires to find the sum of all the distances between the individual pairs of frames along whichever path between the bottom left and top right corners in Fig. 7.3 that gives the smallest distance. This definition will ensure that corresponding frames of similar words are correctly aligned.

One way of calculating this total distance is to consider all possible paths, and add the values of $d(i,j)$ along each one. The distance measure between the patterns is then taken to be the lowest value obtained for the cumulative distance. Although this method is bound to give the correct answer, the number of valid paths becomes so large that the computation is impossible for any practical speech recognition machine. Dynamic programming is a mathematical technique which guarantees to find the cumulative distance along the optimum path without having to calculate the distance along all possible paths.

Let us assume that valid paths obey certain common-sense constraints, such that portions of words do not match when mutually reversed in time (i.e. the path on Fig. 7.3 always goes forward with a non-negative slope). Although skipping single frames could be reasonable in some circumstances, it simplifies the explanation if, for the present, we also assume that we can never omit from the comparison process any frame from either word. In Fig. 7.3, consider a point i,j somewhere in the middle of both words. If this point is on the optimum path then the constraints of the path necessitate that the immediately preceding point on the path is $i-1,j$ or $i-1,j-1$ or $i,j-1$. These three points are associated with a horizontal, diagonal or vertical path step respectively. Let $D(i,j)$ be the cumulative distance along the optimum path from the beginning of the word to point i,j.

$$D(i,j) = \sum_{\substack{x,y=1,1 \\ \text{along the} \\ \text{best path}}}^{i,j} d(x,y) \tag{7.2}$$

As there are only the three possibilities for the point before point i,j it follows that

$$D(i,j) = \min\left(D(i-1,j),\ D(i-1,j-1),\ D(i,j-1)\right) + d(i,j) \tag{7.3}$$

The value of $D(1,1)$ must be equal to $d(1,1)$ as this point is the beginning of all possible paths. To reach points along the bottom and the left hand side of Fig. 7.3 there is only one possible direction (horizontal or vertical, respectively) so starting with the value of $D(1,1)$ values of $D(i,1)$ or values of $D(1,j)$ can be calculated in turn for increasing values of i or j. Let us assume that we calculate the vertical column, $D(1,j)$, using a reduced form of eqn (7.3) that does not have to consider values of $D(i-1,j)$ or $D(i-1,j-1)$. (As the scheme is symmetrical we could equally well have chosen the horizontal direction instead.) When the first column of values for $D(1,j)$ are known, eqn (7.3) can be applied successively to calculate $D(i,j)$ for columns 2 to n. The value obtained for $D(n,N)$ is the score for the best way of matching the two words. For simple speech recognition applications, only the final score is required, and the only working memory needed during the calculation is a one-dimensional array for holding a column (or row) of $D(i,j)$ values. However, there will then be no record at the end of what the optimum path was, and if this information is required for any purpose it is also necessary to store a two-dimensional array of back-pointers, which indicate which direction was chosen at each stage. It is not possible to know until the end has been reached whether any particular point will lie on the optimum path, and this information can only be found by tracing back from the end.

7.6 REFINEMENTS TO ISOLATED WORD DP MATCHING

The algorithm represented by eqn (7.3) is intended to deal with variations of time scale between two otherwise similar words. However, if two examples of a word have the same length but one is faster at the beginning and slower at the end, there will be more horizontal and vertical steps in the optimum path and less diagonals. As a result there will be a greater number of values of $d(i,j)$ in the final score for words with time-scale differences than when the time scales are the same. Although it may be justified to have some penalty for time-scale distortion, on the grounds that a word with a very different time scale is more likely to be the wrong word, it is better to choose values of such penalties explicitly than to have them as an incidental consequence of the algorithm. Making the number of contributions of $d(i,j)$ to $D(n,N)$ independent of the path can be achieved by modifying eqn (7.3) to add twice the value of $d(i,j)$ when the path is diagonal. One can then add an independently chosen penalty to the right hand side of eqn (7.3) when the step is either vertical or horizontal. Equation (7.3) then changes to:

$$(7.4)$$

$$D(i,j) = \min\ (D(i-1,j)+d(i,j)+\text{hdp}, D(i-1,j-1)+2d(i,j), D(i,j-1)+d(i,j)+\text{vdp})$$

A suitable value for the horizontal and vertical distortion penalties, hdp and vdp, would probably have to be found by experiment in association with the chosen distance metric. However, it is obvious that, all other things being equal, paths with appreciable time-scale distortion should be given a worse score than diagonal paths, and so the values of the penalties should certainly not be zero.

Even eqn (7.4) will tend to give lower cumulative distances with short templates and higher distances with long templates. The ultimate best-match decision will as a result favour shorter words. This bias can be avoided by dividing the cumulative distance by the length of the template.

The algorithm described above is inherently symmetrical, and so makes no distinction between the word in the store of templates and the new word to be identified. Dynamic programming is, in fact, a much more general technique that can be applied to finding optimum paths for a wide range of applications, and the number of choices at each stage is not restricted to three, as in the example given in Fig. 7.3. Nor is it necessary in speech recognition applications to assume that the best path should include all frames of both patterns. If the properties of the speech only change slowly compared with the frame interval, it is permissible to skip occasional frames, so achieving time-scale compression of the pattern. A particularly useful alternative version of the algorithm is asymmetrical, in that vertical paths are not permitted. The steps have a slope of zero (horizontal), one (diagonal) or two (which skips one frame in the template). Each input frame then makes just one contribution to the total distance, so it is not appropriate to double the distance contribution for diagonal paths and normalization for template length is not required. Many other variants of the algorithm have been proposed, including one that allows average slopes of 0.5, 1 and 2, in which the 0.5 is achieved by preventing a horizontal step if the previous step was horizontal. Provided the details of the formula are sensibly chosen, all of these algorithms can work well. In a practical implementation computational convenience may be the reason for choosing one in preference to another.

7.7 SCORE PRUNING

Although DP algorithms provide a great computational saving compared with exhaustive search of all possible paths, the remaining computation can be substantial, particularly if each incoming word has to be compared with a large number of candidates for matching. Any possible saving in computation that does not affect the accuracy of the recognition result is therefore desirable. One possible computation saving is to exploit the fact that it is very unlikely, in the calculations for any column on Fig. 7.3, that the best path for a correctly-matching word will pass through any points where the cumulative distance, $D(i,j)$, is much in excess of the lowest value in that column. The saving can be achieved by not allowing paths from badly scoring points to propagate further (sometimes known as **pruning** because the growing paths are like branches of a tree). There will then only be a narrow band of possible paths considered, lying on either side of the best path. If this economy is

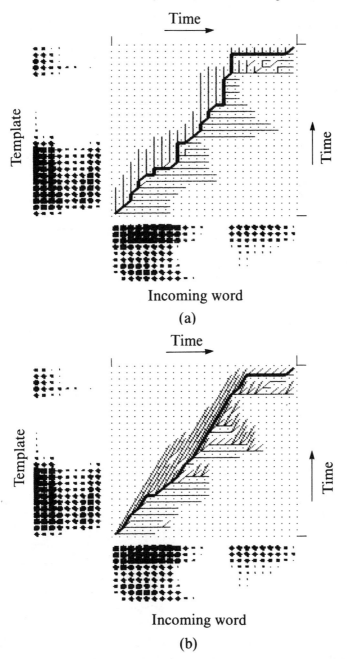

Fig. 7.4(a) DP alignment path between two examples of the word 'eight', with no time-distortion penalty but with score pruning. The optimum path, obtained by tracing back from the top right hand corner, is shown by the thick line. (b) Matching between the same words as in (a), but using the asymmetric algorithm, with slopes of 0, 1 or 2.

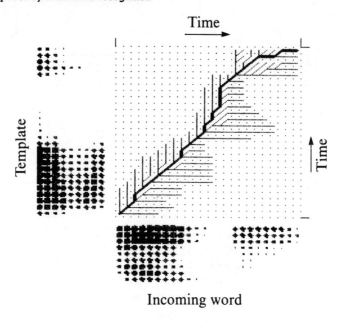

Fig. 7.5   As for Fig. 7.4(a), but with a small time-scale distortion penalty.

applied there can no longer be any guarantee that the DP algorithm will find
the best scoring path. However, with a value of score-pruning threshold that
reduces the average amount of computation by a factor of 5 – 10 the right
path will almost always be obtained where the words are fairly similar. The
only circumstances where this amount of pruning is likely to prevent the
optimum path from being obtained will be if the words are actually different,
when the resultant over-estimate of total distance would not cause any error
in recognition.

   Figs 7.4(a), 7.5 and 7.6 illustrate DP paths using the symmetrical algorithm
for the words illustrated in Figs 7.1 and 7.2. Fig. 7.4(b) shows the
asymmetrical algorithm for comparison, with slopes of 0, 1 and 2. In Fig. 7.4
there is no time-distortion penalty, and Fig. 7.5 with a small distortion
penalty shows a much more plausible matching of the two time scales. The
score pruning used in these figures illustrates the fact that there are low
differences in cumulative distance only along a narrow band around the
optimum path. When time alignment is attempted between dissimilar words,
as in Fig. 7.6, a very irregular path is obtained, with a very poor score. The
score pruning could not be used in this illustration, because the optimum path
would have been pruned off before the end of the word.

Time

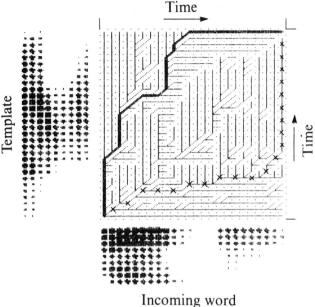

Template

Time

Incoming word

Fig. 7.6 The result of trying to align two dissimilar words ('three' and 'eight') with the same DP algorithm as was used for Fig. 7.5. The score pruning was removed for this illustration because the best path was scoring so badly at the half-way point that it otherwise would not have reached the top right corner. It can be seen that if the template had had its last frame removed the path would have been completely different, as marked with crosses.

7.8 ALLOWING FOR END-POINT ERRORS

Great emphasis has been placed on the problems of end-point detection. If an attempt is made to match two intrinsically similar words in which one has its specified end point significantly in error, the best matching path ought to align all the frames of the two words that really do correspond. Such a path implies that the additional frames of the longer word will all be lumped together at one end, as illustrated in Fig. 7.7. As this extreme time-scale compression is not a result of a genuine difference between the words, it is probably better not to make any time-scale distortion penalty for frames at the ends of the patterns, and with some versions of the algorithm it may be desirable not to add in the values of $d(i,j)$ for the very distorted ends of the path. If the chosen DP algorithm disallows either horizontal steps or vertical steps, correct matching of words with serious end-point errors will not be possible, and with such algorithms it is probably better to remove the path slope constraints just for the end frames.

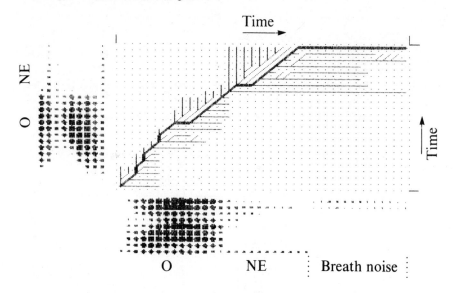

Fig. 7.7 An example of the word 'one', followed by breath noise, being aligned with a 'one' template. A time-scale distortion penalty was used except for the beginning and end frames.

7.9 VARIABLE FRAME RATE ANALYSIS

It has been assumed so far that, once the words have been correctly aligned, all frames are of equal importance in the overall match. However, a slight difference of vowel quality, for example, may not affect the identity of a word, whereas formant transitions at vowel–consonant boundaries may be crucial in identifying the consonant. Because, for many consonants, such transitions are very rapid, they do not occupy many frames. They therefore make only a small contribution to the cumulative distance, even when they match fairly badly. The vowels and steady-state parts of long consonants can, in contrast, make a large contribution to the cumulative distance even when they match fairly well on each frame.

To overcome this difficulty it is necessary to give more weight to parts of the signal that are changing rapidly, and less weight to long steady regions. One way that is sometimes used to achieve this effect is to perform the original acoustic analysis at a high frame rate (e.g. 200 frames per second), but then to discard a variable proportion of the frames depending on the distance between consecutive pairs of frames. Thus all frames are retained in rapid transitions, but perhaps only one in five is kept in very steady long vowels. The cumulative distance of the time-aligned patterns then shows much greater relative sensitivity to mismatch in transition regions.

7.10 EXTENSION OF DYNAMIC PRGRAMMING TO CONNECTED WORDS

Up to now we have assumed that the words to be matched have been spoken in isolation, and their beginnings and ends have therefore already been identified (although perhaps with difficulty). When words are spoken in a normal connected fashion, recognition is much more difficult because it is generally not possible to determine where one word ends and the next one starts independently of identifying what the words are. For example, in the sequence 'six teenagers' it would be difficult to be sure that the first word was 'six' rather than 'sixteen' until the last syllable of the phrase had been spoken, and 'sixty' might also have been a possible choice before the [n] occurred. In some cases, such as the 'grade A' example given in Chapter 1, a genuine ambiguity may remain, but in most limited-vocabulary situations the ambiguities are resolved when at most two or three syllables have followed a word boundary. It is, however, obvious that the simple matching of word patterns between already-specified end points is no longer possible for connected speech.

There is, of course another problem with connected speech as a result of the co-articulation between adjacent words. It is not possible even to claim the existence of a clear point where one word stops and the next one starts. However, the effect of co-articulation mainly affects the ends of words, and apart from a likely speeding up of the time scale, words in a carefully spoken connected sequence do not normally differ drastically from their isolated counterparts except near the ends. In matching connected sequences of words for which separate templates are already available one might thus define the best matching word sequence to be given by the sequence of templates which when joined end to end provides the best match to the input. It is, of course, assumed that the optimum time alignment is used for the sequence, as with DP for isolated words. Although this model of connected speech completely ignores co-articulation, it is successfully used by most existing connected speech recognition products.

As with the isolated-word time-alignment process, there seems to be a potentially explosive increase in computation, as every frame must be considered as a possible boundary between words. When each frame is considered as an end point for one word, all other permitted words in the vocabulary have to be considered as possible starters. Once again the solution to the problem is to apply dynamic programming, but in this case the algorithm is applied to word sequences as well as to frame sequences within words. There are a few possible algorithms that have been developed to extend the isolated-word DP method to work economically across word boundaries. One of the most straightforward is described below.

In Fig. 7.8 consider a point that represents a match between frame i of a multi-word input utterance with frame j of template number k. Let the cumulative distance from the beginning of the utterance along the best-

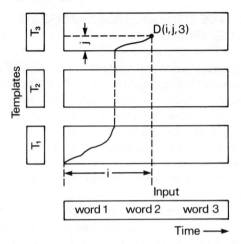

Fig. 7.8 Diagram indicating the best-matching path from the beginning of an utterance to the jth frame of template T_3 and the ith frame of the input. In the example shown the point i is in the middle of the second word of the input, so the best path includes one complete template (T_1) and a part of T_3. The cumulative distance at this point is denoted by $D(i,j,3)$ or, in general as $D(i,j,k)$ for the kth template.

matching sequence of complete templates followed by the first j frames of template k be $D(i,j,k)$. The best path through template k can be found by a similar process to that for isolated word recognition. However, in contrast to the isolated case, it is not known where on the input utterance the match with template k should finish, and for every input frame any valid path that reaches the end of the template k could join to the beginning of the path through another template, representing the next word. As the cumulative distance does not separate the components for individual templates, it is not possible to apply the score normalization by template length that is required for the symmetrical algorithm, and the asymmetrical form is therefore preferred. For each input frame, to find the correct cumulative score to use at the beginning of any new template, m, one must choose the lowest of the cumulative scores achieved for that input frame at the end of all templates that may precede it.

$$D(i, 1,m) = \min_{\text{over } k} (D(i-1,L(k),k)) + d(i,1,m) \qquad (7.5)$$

where $L(k)$ is the length of template k.

The use of $i-1$ in eqn (7.5) implies that moving from the last frame of one template to the first frame of another always involves advancing one frame on the input (i.e. in effect only allowing diagonal paths between templates). This restriction is a consequence of using the asymmetrical DP algorithm, and is also necessary because the scores for the ends of all other templates will not yet be available for input frame i when the path decision has to be made. Of course, a horizontal path from within template m could have been included in eqn (7.5), or paths skipping final frames of the previous template, but they have been omitted to simplify the explanation. A time-scale distortion penalty has not been included for the same reason.

In the same way as for the beginning of isolated words, one can start the process off at the beginning of an utterance because all stored values of $D(0,L(k),k)$ will then be zero.

At the end of an utterance the template that gives the lowest cumulative distance is, of course, assumed to represent the final word of the sequence, but its identity gives no indication of the templates that preceded it. These can only be determined by storing pointers to the preceding templates associated with each path as it evolves, and then tracing back when the final point is reached. If required, it is then also possible to recover the positions in the input sequence where the templates of the matching sequence start and finish, so segmenting the utterance into separate words.

The process as described so far assumes that any utterance can be modelled completely by a sequence of the available templates. In practice a speaker may sometimes pause between words, so producing a period of silence (or background noise) in the middle of an utterance. The same algorithm can still be used for this situation by also storing a template representing a short period of silence, and allowing the **silence template** to be included between appropriate pairs of valid words. If the silence template is also allowed to be chosen at the beginning or end of the sequence the problem of end-point detection is then greatly eased. It is only necessary to choose a threshold that will never be exceeded by the background noise, and, after the utterance has been detected, to extend it by several frames at each end to be sure of including any low-intensity parts of the words. If the word templates do not include any such low-intensity ends the initial and final parts of the utterance presented for matching can then be well modelled by a sequence of one or more silence templates.

It will also often happen when a sequence of words is being spoken that unintentional extraneous noises (such as grunts, coughs, lip smacks, etc.) may be included between words. In an isolated word recognizer these noises will not match well to any of the templates, and can be rejected as a consequence of their poor matching score. In a connected word algorithm there is no provision for not matching any part of the sequence. However, the rejection of these unintentional insertions can be arranged by having a special template, often referred to as a **wildcard template**, that by-passes the usual distance calculation and is deemed to match with any frame of the input to produce a standard value of distance. This value is chosen to be greater than would be expected for corresponding frames of equivalent words, but less than would occur when trying to match quite different sounds. The wildcard will then provide the best-scoring path in attempting to match spurious sounds and words not in the stored vocabulary of templates, but would never be chosen in preference to any of the well-matched words in the input.

7.11 CONTINUOUS RECOGNITION

In the connected word algorithm just described, start and finish points of the input utterance must at least be approximately determined. However, it is not generally necessary to wait till the end of an utterance before identifying the early words. Even before the end, one can trace back along all current paths through the tree that represents the candidates for the template sequence. The structure of this tree is always such as to produce additional branching as time goes forward, but the ends of many of the 'twigs' do not represent a low enough cumulative distance to successfully compete with other twigs as

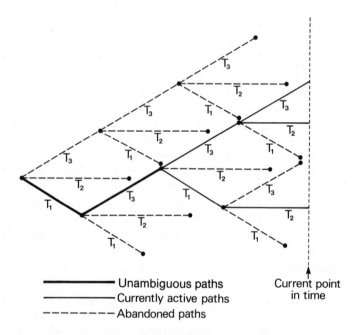

```
————————— Unambiguous paths        Current point
——————— Currently active paths       in time
— — — — — Abandoned paths
```

Fig. 7.9 This diagram illustrates trace-back through the word decision tree to identify unambiguous paths for a three-word vocabulary continuous recognizer. Paths are abandoned where the cumulative distances of all routes to the ends of the corresponding templates are greater than for paths to the ends of different template sequences at the same points in the input. The template sequences still being considered are T_1-T_3-T_3-T_3, T_1-T_3-T_3-T_2 and T_1-T_3-T_1-T_2. It will be noticed that template T_2 is being scored separately for two different preceding sequences.

starting points for further branching, and paths up these twigs are therefore abandoned. It follows that tracing back from all currently active twigs will normally involve coalescence of all these paths into a single 'trunk', which therefore represents a uniquely defined sequence of templates (see Fig. 7.9). The results up to the first point of splitting of active paths can therefore be output from the machine, and once that has been done the back-pointers identifying that part of the path are no longer needed, nor are those representing abandoned paths. The memory used for storing them can therefore be released for re-use in connection with new parts of the input signal.

It is apparent from the above explanation that a recognizer of the type described can operate continuously, with a single pass through the input data, outputting its results always a few templates behind the current best match. The consequent continual increase of cumulative distance as time progresses can be avoided by subtracting the current minimum distance from all of the scores for every input frame. As the scores for all template frames are treated identically, this process does not affect any path decisions. Silence templates are used to match the signal when the speaker pauses, and wildcards are used for extraneous noises or inadmissible words. The time lag for output is determined entirely by the need to resolve ambiguity. Where two alternative sequences of connected words both match the input well, but with different boundary points (such as 'grey day' and 'grade A') it is necessary to reach the end of the ambiguous sequence before a decision can be reached on any part of it. (In the example just given, the decision might even then be wrong because of the inherent ambiguity in the acoustic signal.) On the other hand, if the input matches very badly to all except one of the permitted words, all paths not including that word will be abandoned as soon as the word has finished. In fact, if score pruning is used to cause poor paths to be abandoned early, the path in such a case may be uniquely determined even at a matching point within the word, so enabling the decision on a word to be output before the speaker has finished saying it. There is plenty of evidence that human listeners also often decide on the identity of a long word before it is complete if its beginning is sufficiently distinctive.

7.12 SYNTACTIC CONSTRAINTS

The rules of grammar often prevent certain sequences of words from occurring in human language, and these results apply to particular syntactic classes, such as nouns, verbs, etc. In the more artificial circumstances in which speech recognizers are currently used, the tasks can often be arranged to apply much more severe constraints on which words are permitted to follow each other. Although applying such constraints requires more care in designing the application of the recognizer, it usually offers a substantial gain in recognition accuracy because there are then fewer potentially confusable words to be compared. The incidental saving in computation resulting from reducing the number of templates that need to be matched usually more than compensates for the additional complexity needed to implement the syntactic rules.

7.13 TRAINING A RECOGNIZER

In all the algorithms described in this chapter it is assumed that suitable templates for the words of the vocabulary are available in the machine. Usually the templates must be made from speech of the intended user, and thus a **training session** is required for enrolment of each new user, who is required to give examples of all the vocabulary words. If the same user regularly uses the machine, the templates can be stored in some back-up memory for using each time the recognizer is switched on, and enrolment then merely consists of re-loading the correct set of stored templates. For isolated word recognizers the only technical problem with training is end-point detection. If the templates are stored with wrong end points the error will affect recognition of every subsequent occurrence of the faulty word. Some recognizers try to ensure more reliable templates by time aligning a few examples of each word and averaging the measurements in corresponding frames. This technique gives some protection against occasional end-point errors, because the words then give a poor match in this alignment process and could thus be rejected.

If a system containing a connected word recognition algorithm is available, the templates can be segmented from the surrounding silence by means of a special training syntax, in which only silence and wildcard templates are allowed. The new template candidate will obviously not match the silence, so it will be allocated to the wildcard. The boundaries of the wildcard match will then be taken as the end points of the template word.

In acquiring templates for connected word recognition more realistic training examples can be obtained if connected words are used for the training. Again the recognition algorithm can be used to determine the template end points, but the syntax would have the preceding and following words specified as existing templates, with just the new word to be captured represented by a wildcard between them. Provided the surrounding words can be chosen to give clear acoustic boundaries where they join to the new word, the segmentation will then be fairly accurate. This process is often called **embedded training**.

7.14 SPEAKER-INDEPENDENT RECOGNITION

A recognizer may be required to be used by a wide variety of speakers without re-training. In this case the templates available must be representative of the speech of any of the expected speakers, and so several templates must be provided for each word. The usual method of constructing such templates is to collect many utterances of the vocabulary words spoken by a wide variety of speakers. The resultant word patterns are then aligned with each other so that each one can be represented by a single point in the same multi-dimensional feature-by-time space. These points are then clustered into a fairly small number of groups that are chosen to represent the spread of the word patterns in the space. Templates are then made to represent the average properties in each cluster.

During recognition, any valid incoming vocabulary word can be expected to match reasonably well with one of the templates. However, the dis-criminating power of such a machine must be less than an equivalent machine trained for a single speaker. The clustered templates are not likely to be such a good match for any particular speaker, and there is a much greater chance that one of the several alternative templates available for competing words will yield a smaller cumulative distance. In practical recognizers the difference in performance is usually accommodated by using much smaller vocabularies in speaker-independent mode.

Speaker-independent recognizers of the type just described are able to work just as well when each successive word is spoken by a different speaker. This facility is never normally required for any practical task, so some per-formance improvement should be obtainable by using pre-determined templates initially, but subsequently modifying the set of templates to make it more suitable for the new speaker whenever a word is correctly recognized. Of course, it is vital that adaptation should not take place when the recognition is in error, so some means has to be provided to confirm the recognition results. One possibility is simply to ask the user to confirm the result for each word or phrase by saying one of a very easily recognized pair of response words. An alternative is to design an interactive dialogue for use when a new speaker starts which will ensure that a set of known words must be spoken to start the adaptation process. However, the latter method is not really different in principle from explicitly training the machine for each word of a new user unless it is possible to find systematic transformations that can be derived for a few words and then applied to the whole vocabulary. One straightforward method to achieve this aim would be to disallow all templates that were not derived from the same speakers who provided the data for the first few successful matches achieved.

7.15 THE EFFECTS OF BACKGROUND NOISE

In many recognition tasks background noise in the environment is a serious problem. It has to be accepted that in conditions of high noise it is not possible in principle to distinguish between words that differ only in low-level regions of the spectrum, where they are seriously contaminated by noise.

However, the information for discriminating a limited vocabulary of words is still often available in the acoustic signal, as can be demonstrated by the success of humans when listening to the same noisy material.

If the background noise is high it will normally be impossible to achieve sufficiently reliable end-point detection, and therefore a connected word algorithm will be desirable even for recognizing isolated words. Training would then have to be done separately in the absence of noise.

Unfortunately, if training and recognition are done under different noise conditions, the patterns for the words will not match well because of the corruption of the lower-level parts of the speech spectrum by the noise. However, the higher-level parts of the speech spectrum, in the vicinity of intense formants, are likely to be above the noise level, and will still therefore be a good match to the corresponding parts of the templates.

The best use of the available information can be obtained if a new distance metric is used, which gives proper weight to those feature differences which are reliable, but which ignores differences where noise corruption prevents one from knowing whether there is really a difference in the underlying speech. Provided the acoustic analysis does not mix noise-corrupted and reliable parts of the signal into the same features (e.g. filter-bank analysis is suitable) it is not difficult to design distance metrics with the right properties. It is necessary to have an estimate of the current noise level in each spectral channel, which could be collected in intervals between utterances. For each feature of each frame a decision can then be made whether it is significantly above the noise, and therefore probably genuine, or whether it may be a consequence of noise alone. When an input feature is not significantly above the noise level, it is not possible to know the true level of the underlying speech. However, if this feature is being compared with a template feature well above the noise level, it is known that the true distance between the two features must be at least the measured distance between the template and the noisy input. Therefore the measured value should be added to the cumulative distance. When a template feature is of lower level than a noisy input feature there is no evidence that there is any difference in the underlying speech, and the distance contribution should therefore be zero.

SUMMARY
Chapter 7

Most current speech recognition machines work by pattern matching on whole words. Acoustic analysis, for example by a bank of band-pass filters, describes the speech as a sequence of feature vectors, which are compared with stored templates for all the words in the vocabulary using a suitable distance metric. Matching is improved if speech level is coded logarithmically and level variations are normalized. Other analysis methods include linear prediction analysis and methods based on models of auditory perception.

Two major problems with isolated word recognition are end-point detection and time-scale variation. The time-scale problem can be overcome by using dynamic programming to find the best way of aligning the time scales of the incoming word and each template (known as dynamic time warping). Performance is improved by the use of penalties for time-scale distortion. Score pruning, which abandons alignment paths that are scoring badly, can save a lot of computation. Greater relative weight to phonetically important transitions can be given by using variable frame rate analysis.

Dynamic programming can be extended to deal with sequences of connected words, and to operate continuously, outputting words a second or two after they have been spoken. A wildcard template can be provided to cope with extraneous noises and words that are not in the vocabulary.

A syntax is often provided to prevent illegal sequences of words from being recognized. This method increases accuracy and reduces the computation.

Recognizers are usually 'trained' by giving them examples of all words from the intended user. Sometimes the training is done using several talkers and several templates per word to provide speaker-independent recognition

It is possible to reduce errors caused by background noise by modifying the distance metric so that it only uses information in the speech spectrum that is above the noise level, and therefore reliable.

EXERCISES
Chapter 7

E7.1 Give examples of factors which will cause acoustic differences between utterances of the same word. Why does simple pattern matching work reasonably well in spite of this variability?

E7.2 What are the reasons in favour of logarithmic representation of power in filter-bank analysis? What difficulties can arise as a result of the logarithmic scale.?

E7.3 What are the advantages and disadvantages of orthogonal transformations (such as the cosine transform) when applied to spectral cross-sections?

E7.4 Explain the principles behind dynamic time warping, illustrated by a simple diagram.

E7.5 Describe the special precautions which are necessary when using the symmetrical DTW algorithm for isolated word recognition.

E7.6 How can a DTW isolated-word recognizer be made more tolerant of end-point errors?

E7.7 Why is the symmetrical DP algorithm less suitable for connected-word recognition?

E7.8 How can a connected-word recognizer be used to segment a speech signal into individual words?

E7.9 What extra processes are needed to turn a connected-word recognizer into a continuous recognizer?

E7.10 Describe a training technique suitable for connected-word recognizers.

8

STOCHASTIC MODELS FOR WORD RECOGNITION

8.1 ALLOWING FOR FEATURE VARIABILITY IN PATTERN MATCHING

The recognition methods described in the previous chapter exploit the fact that repeated utterances of the same word normally have more similar acoustic patterns than utterances of different words. However, it is to be expected that some parts of a pattern may vary more from occurrence to occurrence than do other parts. In the case of connected words, the ends of the template representing each word are likely to have a very variable degree of match, depending on the amount that the input pattern is modified by co-articulation with the particular words that are adjacent. There is also no reason to assume that the individual features of the feature vector that represents any one frame are of equal consistency. In fact, it may well occur that the value of a particular feature may be quite critical at a particular frame of one word, and yet it may be very variable and therefore not significant in some part of a different word.

Time-scale variability was also discussed in Chapter 7. It must always be desirable to have some penalty for time-scale distortion, as durations of speech sounds are not normally wildly different between different occurrences of the same word. However, there is no reason to assume the time distortion penalty should be constant for all parts of all words. For example, it is known that long vowels can vary in length a lot, whereas most spectral transitions associated with consonants only change in duration comparatively slightly.

From the above discussion it can be seen that the ability of a recognizer to distinguish between words is likely to be improved if the variability of the patterns can be taken into account. We should not penalize the matching of a particular word if the parts that match badly are parts which are known to vary extensively from utterance to utterance. However, to use information about variability properly we have to have some way of collecting statistics which represent the variability of the word patterns, and some way of using this variability in the pattern-matching process.

If we wish to use information about variability to improve recognition of whole words we will need to determine the statistics of the variation shown by many examples of each word pattern for a representative range of conditions under which the recognizer will be used. If we have a connected word recognizer, the range of conditions must, of course, include a representative range of preceding and following words, so that variation arising from word-boundary co-articulation can be included. We could associate corresponding parts of different examples of a word by using dynamic programming to achieve time alignment. In the time-alignment process the frame numbers should be changed where necessary so that corresponding frames in all examples are given the same frame numbers. It would then be possible to calculate the mean and standard deviation for each feature of each frame of the aligned words, using the standard statistical formulae:

$$\mu_{jk} = \frac{1}{W} \sum_{w=1}^{W} f_{jkw} \tag{8.1}$$

$$\sigma_{jk}^2 = \frac{1}{W} \sum_{w=1}^{W} (f_{jkw} - \mu_{jk})^2 \tag{8.2}$$

where W is the number of training examples, f_{jkw} is the value of the kth feature of frame number j in the time-aligned version of the wth occurrence of the word, μ_{jk} is the mean, σ_{jk} is the standard deviation and σ_{jk}^2 is the variance.

An intuitively attractive way of introducing feature variability into a squared Euclidean distance metric for ASR might be by dividing each difference from the mean template value by the associated standard deviation:

$$d_j = \sum_{k=1}^{n} \left(\frac{f_k - \mu_{jk}}{\sigma_{jk}} \right)^2 \tag{8.3}$$

where d_j is the distance from frame j of the average time-aligned training words, f_k is the kth feature of the input frame being considered and n is the number of features in one feature vector.

Although eqn (8.3) is a straightfoward way of allowing for variability of features in the Euclidean distance calculation, it does not take into account the fact that there will often be substantial correlation between the variations of different features in the feature vectors. A particular case is the correlation related to variations in speech level, mentioned in section 7.2.2. It is also obviously desirable to have a mathematical basis for choosing time-distortion penalties – in particular to make them of appropriate size for each separate part of a word. However, refinements to overcome these difficulties will not be considered until we have introduced a completely different way of defining the degree of fit between a word and the training data, as an alternative to cumulative distance.

8.2 INTRODUCTION TO HIDDEN MARKOV MODELS

Up to now we have considered choosing the best matching word on the basis of finding the template which gives the minimum cumulative distance along the optimum matching path, where feature variability is taken into account to scale the distance measurements. An alternative approach is, for each possible word, to postulate some device, or **model**, which can generate patterns of features to represent the word. Every time the model for a particular word is activated, it will produce a set of feature vectors that represents an example of the word and, if the model is a good one, the statistics of a very large number of such sets of feature vectors will be similar to the statistics measured for human utterances of the word. The best matching word in a recognition task can then be defined as being that word whose model is most likely to produce the observed sequence of feature vectors. What we have to calculate for each word is then not a 'distance' from a template, but the *a posteriori* probability that its model could have produced the observed set of feature vectors. We do not actually have to make the model produce the feature vectors, but we use the known properties of each model for the probability calculations.

Of course, if we wish to derive the probability, $p(w \mid 1 \; F)$, of a particular word, w, having been uttered when we observe a set of features, F, we must also take into account the *a priori* probabilities of the possible words (which must by definition sum to 1). For this purpose it is necessary to use Bayes' theorem:

$$p(w|F) = p(F|w).p(w)/p(F) \tag{8.4}$$

This equation states that the probability of the word given the features is equal to the probability of the features given the word, multiplied by the probability of the word irrespective of the features, and divided by the probability of the features. The probability, $p(F)$, of observing a particular set of features, F, does not depend on which word is being considered as a possible match, and therefore only acts as a scaling factor on the probabilities. It can thus be ignored, because it does not affect the choice of word. If for the particular application all permitted words are equally likely, or if we have no information about their relative probabilities, then the $p(w)$

term can also be ignored, so we merely have to choose the word model that maximizes the probability, $p(F|w)$, of producing the feature set, F.

The way we have already represented words as sequences of template frames gives us a starting point for the form of a possible model. Let the model for any word be capable of being in one of a sequence of **states**, each of which can be associated with one or more frames of the input. In general the model moves from one state to another at regular intervals of time equal to the frame interval of the acoustic analysis. However, we know that words can vary in time scale. In the asymmetrical DP algorithm mentioned in Chapter 7 (Fig. 7.4(b), showing a slope of 0, 1 or 2) the time-scale variability is achieved by repeating or skipping frames of the template. In our model this possibility can be represented in the sequence of states by allowing the model to stay in the same state for successive frame times, or to by-pass the next state in the sequence. The form of this simple model is shown graphically in Fig. 8.1. In fact, if a word has a sequence of very similar frames, such as might occur in a long vowel, it is permissible to reduce the number of states in the model by allowing it to stay in the same state for several successive frames. In effect, this repetition occurred on the penultimate template frame of Fig. 7.4(b).

The mathematics associated with a model such as in Fig. 8.1 can be made more tractable if one assumes that the behaviour of the model is a **stochastic** process (i.e. its operation is governed only by a set of probabilities) and that the probabilities of all its alternative actions at any time only depend on the state it is in at that time. The current output of the model is not affected by the sequence of states it passed through earlier to reach its current state, and operation of the model is therefore a first-order Markov process. Although the model structure shown in Fig. 8.1 is quite appropriate for describing words that vary in time scale, the equations that represent the behaviour of the model have exactly the same form even if transitions are allowed between all possible pairs of states in the model.

At every frame time the model is able to change state, and will do so randomly in a way determined by a set of **transition probabilities** associated with the state it is currently in. By definition, the total of all probabilities of all transitions from a state at any frame time must sum to 1, but the sum includes the probability of a transition that re-enters the same state. When the model is

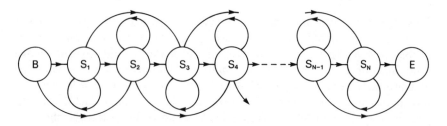

Fig. 8.1   Permitted state transitions for a simple word model.

activated a sequence of feature vectors is emitted, in the same form as sequences of feature vectors that are observed when a word is spoken. However, in the type of model considered here, observing the feature vectors does not completely determine what the state sequence is. In addition to its transition probabilities, each state also has associated with it a probability distribution for the feature vectors. Each probability distribution gives the probability that any set of feature values will be generated when the model is in the associated state. The actual values of features one observes are, therefore, merely probabilistic functions of the states, and the states themselves are hidden from the observer. For this reason this type of model is called a **hidden Markov model** (HMM).

In any implementation of a speech-recognition algorithm, running in some sort of digital computer, the measured features can in practice only have a set of discrete values, even if they are so finely quantized that there is no significant difference from a continuous distribution. Although there are some advantages, which will be considered in section 8.8, in modelling feature probabilities as continuous functions, it will simplify the following explanation if we only consider discrete probability distributions.

8.3 PROBABILITY CALCULATIONS IN HIDDEN MARKOV MODELS

We will start by assuming that some process has already been used to derive the best estimates of the parameters of all the word models. (The procedure for parameter estimation will be discussed later, in sections 8.5 and 8.8.1.) In the recognition process one normally wishes to determine the most likely word, given the observations. As explained in section 8.2, we therefore need to calculate the relative likelihood of each model emitting the observed sequence of features.

A model output representing a whole word arises from the model going through a sequence of states, equal in length to the number of observed feature vectors, N, that represents the word. Let the total number of states in the model be S, and let the identifier for the state that is occupied during any frame, m, of the model's output be s_m. We will also postulate a beginning state, B, and an end state, E, which are not associated with any emitted feature vector, so that it is possible to specify transition probabilities from the start to all permitted first states of the model, and from all possible last emitting states to the end of the word. The probability of a given model producing the observed sequence of feature vectors, F_1 to F_N, is then obtained by summing the probability of each particular state sequence producing the observations, over all possible state sequences of the correct length:

$$p(F_1, F_2, \ldots F_N) = \sum_{\substack{\text{over all} \\ \text{possible state} \\ \text{sequences of} \\ \text{length } N}} p(F_1, F_2, \ldots F_N, s_1, s_2, \ldots s_N)$$

$$p(A \cap B) = p(A|B) \cdot p(B)$$

$$= \sum_{\substack{\text{over all} \\ \text{possible state} \\ \text{sequences of} \\ \text{length } N}} p(F_1, F_2, \ldots F_N | s_1, s_2, \ldots s_N) \cdot p(s_1, s_2, \ldots s_N) \quad (8.5)$$

But the probability of any particular state sequence is given by the product of the transition probabilities:

$$p(s_1, s_2, \ldots s_N) = t_{Bs_1} \cdot \left(\prod_{m=1}^{N-1} t_{s_m s_{m+1}} \right) \cdot t_{s_N E} \quad (8.6)$$

where $t_{s_m s_{m+1}}$ is the probability of a transition from the state in frame m to the state in frame $m+1$; t_{Bs_1} and $t_{s_N E}$ similarly define the transition probabilities from and to the beginning and end states. If we assume that the observed feature vectors are generated independently for each state, the probability of a given state sequence producing the observed features is the product of the individual feature vector probabilities for the specified states:

$$p(F_1, F_2, \ldots F_N | s_1, s_2, \ldots s_N) = \prod_{m=1}^{N} p(F_m | s_m) \quad (8.7)$$

Thus the probability of the model emitting the complete observation sequence is given by:

$$p(F_1, F_2, \ldots F_N) = \sum_{\substack{\text{over all} \\ \text{possible state} \\ \text{sequences of} \\ \text{length } N}} t_{Bs_1} \cdot \left(\prod_{m=1}^{N-1} t_{s_m s_{m+1}} \cdot p(F_m | s_m) \right) \cdot p(F_N | s_N) \cdot t_{s_N E} \quad (8.8)$$

Unless the model has a very small number of states, there will be an astronomical number of possible state sequences, and it would be completely impractical to make the calculations of eqn (8.8) directly for all sequences. One can, however, compute the probability indirectly by using a recurrence relationship. We will use the symbol $p^+(m,j)$ to be the probability of the model being in the jth state after having produced the first m observed feature vectors; the reason for using the plus sign in the notation is not important at this stage, but will be explained in section 8.5.1. The recurrence can be computed in terms of the values of $p^+(m-1,i)$ for all possible previous states, i.

$$p^+(m, j) = p(F_1, F_2, \ldots F_m \text{ and } s_m = j) \tag{8.9}$$

$$= \left(\sum_{i=1}^{S} p^+(m-1, i) . t_{ij} \right) . p(F_m | j) \tag{8.10}$$

The value of $p^+(1,j)$ is the probability of getting the first feature vector from state j, and uses the transition probability, t_{Bj} from the beginning state, B.

$$p^+(1, j) = t_{Bj} . p(F_1 | j) \tag{8.11}$$

The value of $p^+(N,j)$, for the last of the sequence of emitting states, can thus be computed by repeated applications of eqn (8.10) starting from the result of eqn (8.11).

The total probability of the complete set of observations produced by the model must include the transition probabilities into the end state E, and is given by:

$$p(F_1, F_2, \ldots F_N) = \sum_{i=1}^{S} p^+(N, i) . t_{iE} \tag{8.12}$$

Equation (8.12) gives the probability of the model generating the observed data, taking into account all possible sequences of states. If the model can be considered to be a good representation of the word, this quantity may be converted to the relative likelihood of that word having been spoken by application of the Bayes formula given in eqn (8.4).

The total amount of computation needed for all the stages leading up to eqn (8.12) is still substantial, particularly if the model has a large number of states. In general the equations allow transitions to take place between all available pairs of states. However, particularly if the states correspond roughly to successive groups of frames of word templates, as suggested in section 8.2, there should obviously be quite severe constraints on state order. The type of model depicted in Fig. 8.1 allows transitions from each state to only two other states in addition to the self-transition. Any transitions can be disallowed by making the associated transition probabilities equal to zero, and reducing the number of allowed transitions reduces the computational load.

8.4 THE VITERBI ALGORITHM

The probability of the observations, given the model, is made up of contributions from a very large number of alternative state sequences. However, the probability distributions associated with the states will be such that the probability of the observed feature vectors having been produced by many of those states will be microscopically small compared with the probabilities associated with other states. The contribution of the less likely state sequences to the total will thus be very small and, if the feature vector probability distributions of all states are substantially different from each other, the probability of the observations arising from the most likely of all the alternative sequences may not be greatly less than the total probability given by the sum over all possible sequences.

The difference between the total probability and the probability of the most likely sequence will, however, be quite large if the best path includes several consecutive frames shared between a group of two or more states which, although separately identified, have very similar probability distributions for the feature vectors. In such a case the probability of generating the observed feature vectors would be almost independent of how the model distributed its time between the states in this group. The total probability, which is the sum over all possible allocations of frames to states, would then be many times the probability given by the most likely sequence. This point will be considered again in section 8.9. In spite of the theoretical disadvantage of using only the maximum-likelihood path, there can, however, be important computational advantages, and quite good recognition results can be obtained with this method.

The probability of the most likely sequence of states can be calculated by the **Viterbi algorithm** (Viterbi, 1967), which is a dynamic programming algorithm applied to probabilities, rather than to 'distances' as in Chapter 7. Equation (8.5) can be reformulated to give the probability of the observations being given by the most likely sequence of states:

$$\hat{p}(F_1, F_2, \dots F_N) = \begin{array}{c} \text{max. over} \\ \text{all possible} \\ \text{state sequences} \\ \text{of length } N \end{array} \left\{ p(F_1, F_2, \dots F_N, s_1, s_2, \dots s_N) \right\} \quad (8.13)$$

Let us define a new probability, $\hat{p}^*(m,j)$, which is the probability of being in the jth state, after having emitted the first m feature vectors and having been through the most likely sequence of $m-1$ preceding states in the process. Again we have a recurrence relation, equivalent to eqn (8.10):

$$\hat{p}^+(m, j) = \begin{array}{c} \text{max.} \\ \text{over } i \end{array} \left\{ \hat{p}^+(m-1, i).t_{ij} \right\}.p(F_m|j) \quad (8.14)$$

But the conditions for the first state are the same as for the total probability, which was given in eqn (8.11):

$$\hat{p}^+(1, j) = p^+(1, j) = t_{Bj} . p(F_1 | j) \qquad (8.15)$$

Successive applications of eqn (8.14) eventually yield the values for $\hat{p}^+(N,j)$. The probability for the full set of observations being given by the most likely sequence of states is then:

$$\hat{p}(F_1, F_2, \ldots F_N) = \max_{\text{over } i} \left\{ \hat{p}^+(N, i) . t_{iE} \right\} \qquad (8.16)$$

In contrast to eqn (8.12), the operations which lead up to eqn (8.16) contain only products, and no summations. It would make the computation easier if we could replace the multiplications by additions, which can be done be representing all the numbers as logarithms. The conditions for maximizing the right hand side can be achieved by maximizing its logarithm because the logarithmic function is monotonic and increasing. As all probabilities are less than 1, and therefore have negative logarithms, it will tidy the computation a little if we negate each term. We can then find the most likely state sequence by minimizing the resultant expression. Representing $-\ln(\hat{p}^+(m,j))$ by $\hat{P}^+(m,j)$, $-\ln(t_{ij})$ by T_{ij} and $-\ln(p(F_m|j))$ by $P(F_m|j)$, we can replace eqn (8.14) by:

$$\hat{P}^+(m, j) = \min_{\text{over } i} \left\{ \hat{P}^+(m-1, i) + T_{ij} \right\} + P(F_m | j) \qquad (8.17)$$

If the model parameters are known, the quantities $-\ln(t_{ij})$ and $-\ln(p(F_m|j))$ are fixed for given values of i, j and m, and thus in principle the logarithms only need to be calculated once and stored in the machine. The dynamic programming algorithm then only involves summations and comparisons, with no multiplications, and so the computational load is reduced in comparison with the total probability calculation.

8.5 PARAMETER ESTIMATION FOR HIDDEN MARKOV MODELS

In the probability calculations we have considered so far we have assumed that the parameters of the word models, i.e. the transition probabilities and the feature probability distributions for all the states, are already set to their optimum values for modelling the statistics of a very large number of human utterances of all the words that are to be recognized. In the discussion which follows, we will consider the problem of deriving suitable values for these parameters from a quantity of 'training data'. We will assume for the moment that the body of training data is of sufficient size to represent the statistics of the underlying population of possible utterances, and that we have sufficient computational capacity to perform the necessary operations.

Although it is possible to formulate various heuristic methods of analyzing the training data to give rough estimates of suitable parameters for the model, there is no method of calculating the optimum values directly. If, however, one has a set of rough estimates for all parameters it is possible to use their values in equations which will give new estimates for each parameter. It has been proved by Baum (1972) that these new estimates always produce a model that is at least as good as the old one in representing the data, and in general the new estimates give an improved model. If we iterate these equations a sufficiently large number of times the model will then obviously converge to a locally optimum solution. In the re-estimation equations we will use a bar above the symbol to represent a re-estimated value, and the same symbol without the bar to indicate its previous value.

Unfortunately there is no guarantee that this re-estimation will give a global optimum, but with suitable values of starting estimates good models are usually obtained. This aspect will be considered again after the re-estimation equations have been derived.

8.5.1 Forward and backward probabilities

In eqn (8.10), we showed how to compute $p^+(m,j)$, the probability of being in state j after having emitted the first m observed feature vectors. The values of $p^+(m,j)$ must be computed for successive frames in order, going forward from the beginning of the utterance. By exactly the same reasoning we can compute $p^-(m,i)$, which is the **backward** probability of emitting the remaining $N-m$ observed vectors that are needed to make up the complete word, given that the ith state is occupied for frame m. This time the recurrence relationship is in terms of the values of $p^-(m+1,j)$s for all states:

$$p^-(m, i) = p(F_{m+1}, F_{m+2}, \ldots F_N | S_m = i) \tag{8.18}$$

$$= \sum_{j=1}^{S} p^-(m+1, j) . t_{ij} . p(F_{m+1} | j) \tag{8.19}$$

The slight difference in form between the definitions of $p^+(m,j)$ and $p^-(m,i)$ and between eqns (8.9) and (8.18) is necessary because of the way we will combine these quantities in eqn (8.21).

It is necessary for the backward probabilities to start applying the recurrence from the end of the word, and to work backwards through the sequence of frames. The first application of eqn (8.19) uses the fact that the model must be in the end state, E, when the word has finished. All features will then have been emitted, so the value of $p^-(N,i)$ is merely the probability of a transition from state i to the final state:

$$p^-(N, i) = t_{iE} \tag{8.20}$$

The probability of the model being in the ith state for the mth observed frame and of emitting the full set of N feature vectors, must be the product of the forward and backward probabilities:

$$p^*(m, i) = p^+(m, i).p^-(m, i) \tag{8.21}$$

As $p^*(m,i)$ is the probability of generating the full set of feature vectors and being in state i at time m, the probability of the observations irrespective of which state is occupied in frame m must be the sum of $p^*(m,i)$ over all states. The resultant eqn (8.22) is true for any value of the frame number, m.

$$p(F_1, F_2, \ldots F_N) = \sum_{i=1}^{S} p^*(m, i) \tag{8.22}$$

Equation (8.12) is thus merely a special case of eqn (8.22), where $m=N$.

The probability of the model emitting the full set of observed feature vectors and being in state i, irrespective of the frame being considered, is the average of $p^*(m,i)$ over all frames of the word.

$$p^*(i) = \frac{1}{N} \sum_{m=1}^{N} p^*(m, i) \tag{8.23}$$

Equation (8.21) can be extended to compute the probability of the model emitting all the feature vectors, being in state i for frame m and being in state j for frame $m+1$. The computation uses the forward probability for frame m and the backward probability for frame $m+1$, combined with the transition probability, t_{ij}, of moving from i to state j and the probability of state j emitting feature vector F_{m+1}.

$$p^t(m, i, j) = p^+(m, i).p^-(m+1, j).t_{ij}.p(F_{m+1}|j) \tag{8.24}$$

We can use eqn (8.24) to find the probability of producing a transition from state i to state j independent of frame time. We need to average eqn (8.24) over all frames except for the final one, which cannot produce a transition to another emitting state.

$$p^t(i, j) = \frac{1}{N-1} \sum_{m=1}^{N-1} p^t(m, i, j) \tag{8.25}$$

If we had only one example of the word available, we could re-estimate the transition probability, t_{ij}, of the model reaching state j if it is known to be already in state i by dividing eqn (8.25) by a modified form of eqn (8.23), that excludes the final frame of each word.

$$
\bar{t}_{ij} = \frac{\sum\limits_{m=1}^{N-1} p'(m, i, j)}{\sum\limits_{m=1}^{N-1} p^*(m, i)}
\tag{8.26}
$$

In any practical situation there would be several examples of each word, and we need to make a re-estimation taking all of them into account with equal weight. It is not sufficient merely to sum the numerators and denominators of eqn (8.26) over all words, because the current model is likely to fit some example words better than others, and these words would then be given more weight in the re-estimation process. If, however, this effect is corrected by dividing both the numerator and denominator of eqn (8.26) by the probability of generating the features of word w given the current model (denoted by p_w), the overall re-estimation can be performed by extending the operation of eqn (8.26) to include all words. The values of p_w can be derived using eqn (8.12).

$$
\bar{t}_{ij} = \frac{\sum\limits_{w=1}^{W} \frac{1}{p_w} \sum\limits_{m=1}^{N_w-1} p'(m, i, j, w)}{\sum\limits_{w=1}^{W} \frac{1}{p_w} \sum\limits_{m=1}^{N_w-1} p^*(m, i, w)}
\tag{8.27}
$$

where N_w is the number of frames in word w, and $p^*(m,i,w)$ and $p'(m,i,j,w)$ denote the values of $p^*(m,i)$ and $p'(m,i,j)$ respectively for the wth training word.

Simpler formulae for the special cases of t_{Bj} and t_{iE} can also be derived from eqns (8.21) and (8.24).

The probability of observing any feature vector, F_a, when in state i can be similarly derived as the probability of being in state i and observing F_a, divided by the probability of being in state i, again summing over all frames and taking a weighted average over all examples of the word.

$$\bar{p}(F_a|i) = \frac{\displaystyle\sum_{w=1}^{W} \frac{1}{p_w} \sum_{m \ni F_m = F_a} p^*(m, i, w)}{\displaystyle\sum_{w=1}^{W} \frac{1}{p_w} \sum_{m=1}^{N_w} p^*(m, i, w)} \tag{8.28}$$

This use of forward and backward probabilities to re-estimate model parameters is usually known either as the **forward-backward algorithm** or as the **Baum-Welch algorithm** (Baum, 1972).

An equivalent set of formulae can be derived to re-estimate parameters of models using the Viterbi algorithm. In this case Viterbi versions of the forward and backward probabilities, $\hat{p}^+(m,i)$ and $\hat{p}^-(m,i)$ are used in the re-estimation formulae.

8.5.2 Choice of initial values

The goodness of the local optimum derived by the Baum–Welch algorithm depends quite strongly on the initial choices of all the parameters of the model. For example, it can be seen from the derivation of eqn (8.27) from eqn (8.24) that if any of the t_{ij} are given values of zero, their re-estimated values will also always be zero. Setting initial values of some transition probabilities to zero is thus a convenient way of constraining the structure of the word model to prevent it from producing instrinsically implausible state sequences. For example, it would not seem reasonable to allow the model to occupy a state early in the word, and then return to it after having been through several succeeding states. The state sequence in Fig. 8.1 is very constrained, only allowing three non-zero values of t_{ij}, yet is very plausible as a word model.

Within the limitations determined by the chosen model structure, it is desirable to choose the starting values to constrain the model as little as possible. Thus the probability distributions for the features should not be very peaky, and the transition probabilities should not appreciably penalize any permitted paths. Under these conditions it is found that even for very different sets of starting values for the probability distributions and for the between-state transition probabilities, the locally optimum models derived after several iterations of the re-estimation are often very similar. Although all such models will then have states with similar properties, the state identifiers associated with these properties will depend on what parameters were associated with each state at the beginning. The state identifiers may therefore be arbitrarily permuted, unless the state order is very constrained. Unlucky sets of starting values may give rise to a sub-optimum model, but these can in principle be avoided by trying several alternative sets. By testing the results for word discrimination on all the training data, it is then possible to pick the best of the models so derived, but this procedure is computationally very expensive.

If sensible initial guesses for the parameters are based on some heuristic procedure applied to examples of the training data, the models will usually be fairly good to start with and will get close to the local optimum after a very small number of iterations. However, this procedure can be dangerous: for some words the heuristics may make serious errors in interpreting the data, and in these cases the Baum–Welch re-estimation will rapidly converge to a sub-optimal set of parameters.

8.6   CONSEQUENCES OF INSUFFICIENT TRAINING DATA (PART 1)

In the discussion above it is assumed that the data used for training the models contain a large enough number of words for reliable values to be obtained for all the parameters. For any statistical estimation to give sensible results it is obvious that the total number of data items must be significantly larger than the number of separate parameters to be estimated for the distribution. If the number of possible feature vectors is very large, as a result of many possible values for each of several individual features, many feature vectors will not occur at all in a manageable amount of training data. In consequence the generation probabilities for these feature vectors will be estimated as zero. If such a feature vector then occurred in the input during operational use of the recognizer, recognition would not be possible. Two solutions are widely used to overcome this difficulty, as explained below.

8.7   VECTOR QUANTIZATION

The multi-dimensional feature space for any practical method of speech analysis is not uniformly occupied. The types of spectrum cross-section that occur in speech signals cause certain regions of the feature space, corresponding, for example, to the spectra of commonly occurring vowels and fricatives, to be highly used, and other regions to be at most sparsely occupied. It is possible to make a useful approximation to the feature vectors that actually occur by choosing only a small subset (perhaps about 100) of feature vectors, and replacing each measured vector by the one in the subset that is 'nearest' to it according to a suitable distance metric. This process is known as **vector quantization**.

The performance of a vector quantizer depends on the number of different vectors and how they are chosen, but the details of these decisions are outside the scope of this book. It is, however, clear that if a fairly small number of vectors is chosen to represent the well-occupied parts of the feature space, all of the vectors will occur frequently in a training data base of moderate size. It will thus be possible to obtain good estimates of the probability of all feature vectors that are likely to occur for each state of the model.

A fully trained model for a particular word will, of course, have some feature vectors that are given zero probability for all states. For example, the word 'one' would not be expected to contain any examples of a feature vector representing the typical spectrum of an [s] sound. It is, however, important not to allow the probabilities to remain exactly at zero. Otherwise there is the danger of error on an input word that matches fairly well to the properties of one of the models except for just one non-typical frame that is represented by a zero-probability feature vector. In such a case the model will yield zero probability for that sequence of vectors, and the machine will therefore not be able to choose the correct word. Replacing the zero value by a very small number will obviously yield a low probability of generating the observed features for that model, but if the rest of the word is sufficiently distinctive even this low value can be expected to be greater than the probability of generating the same set of features from any of the competing models.

8.8 MULTI-VARIATE CONTINUOUS DISTRIBUTIONS

A more widely used method for coping with the fact that particular sets of finely quantized feature values will occur only very rarely is to represent the distribution of feature vectors by some simple parametric model, and to use the calculated probabilities from this model to supply the probability distributions in the training and recognition processes. The Baum–Welch re-estimation must then be used to optimize the parameters of the feature distribution model, rather than the probabilities of particular feature vectors.

Many natural processes involve variable quantities which approximate reasonably well to the **normal** (or **Gaussian**) distribution. The normal distribution has only two independently specifiable parameters, the mean, μ, and the standard deviation, σ, and the probability density is given by:

$$\phi(x) = \frac{1}{\sigma\sqrt{(2\pi)}} \exp\left(\frac{-(x-\mu)^2}{2\sigma^2}\right) \tag{8.29}$$

When quantities are distributed normally, this simple mathematical description of the distribution makes it possible to calculate the probability of the quantity lying in any range of values provided the mean and standard deviation of the distribution are known.

Of course, many naturally occurring quantities are not normally distributed. For example, speech intensity measured over, say, 20 ms, will certainly not approximate to a normal distribution because it clearly has a hard limit of zero during silences, will be low for much of the time during weak sounds, but will go up to quite high values during more intense vowels. The intensity on a logarithmic scale would have a more symmetrical distribution, which might be nearer to normal, but in this case the low-level end of the distribution will be very dependent on background noise level.

Normal distributions usually fit best to measurements which would be expected to have a preferred value, but where there are various chance factors which can cause deviation from that value. Thus speech features which are derived from the same specific part of a specific word will have a fairly good approximation to a normal distribution. It is therefore very common in speech recognition to assume that feature distributions are normal for each state of a hidden Markov model.

As the features are multi-dimensional, they are assumed to form a multi-variate normal distribution. In general the features may not vary independently, and so their interdependence is specified by a covariance matrix. If the particular form of speech analysis is such that features are substantially uncorrelated, the covariance matrix becomes approximately zero except along its main diagonal, and the probability of a feature vector reduces to a product of probabilities given by the univariate distributions of the separate features.

Let us first consider the probability density, $\phi(F|i)$, where F is a column vector of features, $f_1, f_2, \ldots f_n$. Let M_i be the column vector of means, $\mu_{i1}, \mu_{i2}, \ldots \mu_{in}$, and R_i be the covariance matrix for the distribution of features associated with the ith state. The definition of the multi-variate normal distribution gives the probability density compactly in matrix notation:

$$\phi(F|i) = \frac{1}{|R_i|^{\frac{1}{2}} (2\pi)^{\frac{n}{2}}} \exp\left(\frac{-(F-M_i)^T R_i^{-1} (F-M_i)}{2}\right) \tag{8.30}$$

where $|R_i|$ is the determinant of R_i. In the special case when the features are uncorrelated, eqn (8.30) reduces to the computationally much simpler form:

$$\phi(F|i) = \prod_{k=1}^{n} \frac{1}{\sigma_{ik}\sqrt{(2\pi)}} \exp\left(-\frac{1}{2}\left(\frac{f_k - \mu_{ik}}{\sigma_{ik}}\right)^2\right) \tag{8.31}$$

where f_k is the kth feature of F, μ_{ik} is the mean of the distribution of the k_{th} feature of state i and σ_{ik} is the standard deviation of the kth feature of state i.

The definition of the **probability density function** (p.d.f.), $\phi(x)$, of a variate, x, is such that the probability of an observation lying in an infinitesimal interval of size dx centred on x is $\phi(x)dx$, and is thus infinitesimally small. However, if the continuous probability density functions are used instead of discrete probability distributions in the equations in sections 8.3 – 8.5, the computation will still yield the correct relative likelihoods of the possible observations, as the infinitesimal interval, dx, is common to all likelihood calculations. The probability of observing the features, $p(F)$, independent of which word is spoken, is also affected in the same way by the size of the infinitesimal interval, dx. The probability of the word given the features is therefore still correctly given by eqn (8.4), even if these relative likelihoods are used instead of actual probabilities for $p(F)$ and $p(F|w)$. Although their theoretical interpretations are different, it is thus equally suitable to use either discrete or continuous probability distributions in the calculations of word probability and in the Baum–Welch parameter estimation.

8.8.1 Baum–Welch re-estimation for normal distributions

The means of the p.d.f.s of the features associated with any state can be estimated, as in any calculation of the mean of a statistical distribution, merely by averaging the observed values weighted by their relative frequencies of occurrence. But the frequency of any value occurring in state i is proportional to the probability of the model being in state i when the feature is emitted, given by eqn (8.21). Therefore the re-estimation of feature k when associated with state i is given by:

$$\bar{\mu}_{ik} = \frac{\sum_{w=1}^{W} \frac{1}{p_w} \sum_{m=1}^{N_w} p^*(m, i, w) . f_{kmw}}{\sum_{w=1}^{W} \frac{1}{p_w} \sum_{m=1}^{N_w} p^*(m, i, w)} \tag{8.32}$$

The values in the covariance matrix R_i for state i are given by the standard formula for calculating covariance in multi-variate distributions, again using the probability values for the relative frequencies of occurrence of the deviations from the calculated means:

$$\bar{R}_i = \frac{\sum_{w=1}^{W} \frac{1}{p_w} \sum_{m=1}^{N_w} p^*(m, i, w) . (F_{m,w} - M_i)(F_{m,w} - M_i)^T}{\sum_{w=1}^{W} \frac{1}{p_w} \sum_{m=1}^{N_w} p^*(m, i, w)} \tag{8.33}$$

8.9 DURATION MODELLING IN HIDDEN MARKOV MODELS

The probability of a model staying in the same state, i, for successive frames is

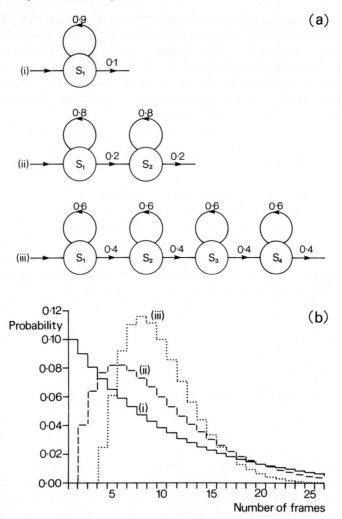

Fig. 8.2(a) Three arrangements of states, each of which has an expected occupation time of 10 frames. (b) Probability of occupancy of groups states in the model sections shown in (a).

determined only by the transition probability, t_{ii}. The expected number of frames it will stay in state i is $1|(1-t_{ii})$, so a value of 0.9 would be appropriate for using one state to model, for example, a steady fricative sound whose expected duration is ten frames. Although the expected total duration in state i in this case is ten frames, the most probable duration is only one frame, which has a probability of 0.1. The probabilities for longer durations decrease exponentially, as shown in trace (i) of Fig. 8.2(b). This distribution of durations is often referred to as a **geometric distribution** because the probabilities for successive numbers of frames form a geometric progression.

Let us assume that the vocabulary contains another word which has a similar sequence of feature vectors but with one of the sounds very much shorter. (An example pair might be 'sin' and 'tin', because the spectrum of a [t] burst is very like that of an [s].) In 'tin' the state corresponding to the [t] burst might have an expected duration of only two frames, which would give a value of 0.5 for t_{ii}. If the feature probability distributions of all the states in the sequence were exactly the same for both words, the probability ratio of a two-frame burst being emitted by the 'sin' model compared with the 'tin' model would only be $(0.9 \times 0.1) : (0.5 \times 0.5)$, which is a ratio of approximately 1 : 3. The effect of this ratio could easily be swamped if there were a small difference in the feature probabilities for the two models, and so the word 'tin' with quite minor difference in articulation would have a high probability of being recognized as 'sin'.

The durational characteristics of first-order Markov models are a major cause of word recognition errors when the number of states is just sufficient to model the significantly different spectral regions of the word. If many more states are available, the Baum–Welch parameter estimation process will normally allocate a group of several states to each long steady region. States within each such group will therefore have similar feature probability distributions, and so alternative paths of any given length through the group will be likely to give similar feature vector sequences. The probability of the path which goes through such a group of states in the minimum number of frames will then be very much lower than the combined probability of all the alternative paths of any substantially greater length. The discrimination of words which differ in length will therefore be much improved.

As explained in section 8.4, the Viterbi interpretation of a word, which only considers the most likely path through a group of states, does not give this benefit from including more states in the model.

Provided the total likelihood interpretation is being used, some of the advantages of the improved time modelling with extra states can in fact be obtained by simply splitting each long duration state into several sub-states with shorter expected durations and all with identical probability distributions for the feature vectors. The relative probabilities of different dwell times within a pair of states where each state has a repeat probability of 0.8 are shown in trace (ii) of Fig. 8.2(b). The expected duration for the pair is ten frames, as for trace (i), but the variation of probability with duration is much more like that expected for speech sounds within a word. An even more realistic time distribution is obtained for four states with a repeat probability of 0.6, as shown in trace (iii) of Fig. 8.2(b).

Many other methods have been proposed for improving the duration characteristics of hidden Markov models, including some that model duration distributions of each state explicitly. The performance of such methods can be very good, but usually at the expense of considerably more computation and a greater number of model parameters to be estimated.

8.10 USE OF NORMAL DISTRIBUTIONS WITH THE VITERBI ALGORITHM

It was explained in section 8.4 that there are advantages in using negated logarithms when calculating the maximum-likelihood state sequence using the Viterbi algorithm. In the case of a set of uncorrelated normal distributions for the features, the negative of the log probability density of any of the feature values can be calculated by taking logarithms of eqn (8.29):

$$-\ln(\phi(x)) = \frac{1}{2}\ln(2\pi) + \ln(\sigma) + \frac{1}{2}\left(\frac{x-\mu}{\sigma}\right)^2 \qquad (8.34)$$

The negative log probability density of a complete vector of n features for state i is therefore:

$$-\ln(\phi(F|i)) = \frac{n}{2}\ln(2\pi) + \sum_{k=1}^{n}\ln(\sigma_{ik}) + \frac{1}{2}\sum_{k=1}^{n}\left(\frac{f_k - \mu_{ik}}{\sigma_{ik}}\right)^2 \qquad (8.35)$$

The Viterbi calculation of eqn (8.17) then becomes

$$\hat{P}^+(m, j) = \min_{\text{over } i}\left\{\hat{P}^+(m-1, i) + T_{ij}\right\} + \frac{n}{2}\ln(2\pi) + \sum_{k=1}^{n}\ln(\sigma_{jk})$$
$$+ \frac{1}{2}\sum_{k=1}^{n}\left(\frac{f_k - \mu_{jk}}{\sigma_{jk}}\right)^2 \qquad (8.36)$$

The term $\frac{n}{2}\ln(2\pi)$ is a constant, which will scale the calculated likelihood but will not affect the choice of optimal state sequence. The value of $\sum_{k=1}^{n}\ln(\sigma_{jk})$ depends on the state, but is independent of the observed feature values. The term $\sum_{k=1}^{n}\left(\frac{f_k - \mu_{jk}}{\sigma_{jk}}\right)^2$ can be recognized as simply the square of the scaled Euclidean distance between the observed features and the feature means for template frame j, as given near the beginning of this chapter in eqn (8.3).

It is interesting to compare the Markov probability calculation with the cumulative distance formula for a simple asymmetric dynamic programming algorithm in which each input frame occurs exactly once in the distance calculation. If the DP uses a squared Euclidean distance metric, it can be regarded as a special case of a hidden Markov algorithm, in which the word models have one state per template frame, and the features are assumed to be normally distributed with unit variance. In these circumstances the $\sum_{k=1}^{n}\ln(\sigma_{jk})$ term of eqn (8.36) becomes zero, and the T_{ij} terms can be regarded as representing the time distortion penalties. Where only slopes of 0, 1 and 2 are permitted, as for Fig. 8.1, the time distortion penalties for other values of slope are $-\ln(0)$, and are therefore infinite.

Although the T_{ij} terms represent the time distortion penalties, it would be wrong to assume that the distortion penalties for DP template matching should be set by Baum–Welch re-estimation even if sufficient training data were available to get statistically reliable values. Because of the duration modelling weaknesses of the Viterbi algorithm described in the previous section, such penalties could be far too small in long steady sounds. With only a small amount of training data, there is a serious danger of under-training, explained in section 8.12. If constant distortion penalties are acceptable it is easy to set them by experiment, plotting the alignment paths and assessing them for plausibility, as suggested in Chapter 7.

8.11 PRACTICAL PROBLEMS OF COMPUTATION

The calculation of the forward and backward probabilities of particular sequences of features involves multiplication of a very large number of probability components, most of which are much less than 1. The results are in general likely to have very low values, and mostly will be much smaller than the minimum size of floating point number that can be held in any normal computer. In the case of the Viterbi calculations, the range can be compressed sufficiently by taking logarithms, but for total likelihood calculations the need to also perform summations appears to preclude this possibility.

The usual solution to the number range problem is to check the size of the probabilities at each stage of the recursion, and to multiply the results by a scale factor that will bring the numbers back into the centre of the available range. It is possible to use a scaling technique such that the product of the scale factors is equal to $1/p_w$. The use of this scaling enables the $1/p_w$ terms to be omitted from the Baum–Welch re-estimation formulae for multiple training utterances. However, scale factors must be noted and taken into account in estimating the relative likelihoods that any set of feature vectors has been generated by each word model. As the product of the scale factors will usually exceed the permitted number range it is necessary to represent it logarithmically, by adding the logarithms of the individual scale factors.

The need for scaling could be avoided by logarithmic representation of the numbers if the additions needed for the forward and backward probabilities could be made while the numbers were still in their logarithmic form. Fortunately a method of adding numbers when they are coded logarithmically has been described by Kingsbury and Rayner (1971) for a completely different purpose.

Let A and B be two positive numbers represented in a computer only as $\ln A$ and $\ln B$. Consider the problem of deriving $\ln(A+B)$ without taking antilogs of the given numbers. It is obvious that:

$$A+B = A(1+B|A) \tag{8.37}$$

Therefore

$$\ln(A+B) = \ln(A(1+B/A)) = \ln A + \ln(1+B/A) \qquad (8.38)$$

Let us assume that we have ordered the numbers A and B so that $A \geqslant B$. It then follows that $1 \leqslant 1 + B = A \leqslant 2$. If $\ln (A+B)$ is required with only moderate accuracy, very small values of B/A can be replaced by zero without causing a significant error. For example, a 1% accuracy for $A+B$ would enable values of B/A less than 0.01 to be ignored. The values of $\ln(1+ B/A)$ for larger values of B/A can be found with sufficient accuracy in terms of $\ln(B/A)$ by means of a pre-computed look-up table. The form of the function to be tabulated is shown in Fig. 8.3 for a range of B/A from 0.01 to 1. If an error of 0.01 in the result is acceptable (roughly 1% error in $A + B$) the table only needs entries for 115 equally spaced values of $\ln(B/A)$.

The procedure for finding $\ln(A + B)$ is as follows:

1　If $\ln B > \ln A$ then transpose $\ln A$ and $\ln B$.
2　Find $\ln (B/A)$ by forming $\ln B - \ln A$.
3　Use the result of **2** to select a value from the look-up table.
4　Add the result of **3** to $\ln A$.

If the above method is implemented using a suitable scale factor for the logarithms, it is then possible to make all the necessary probability calculations for recognition using integer arithmetic on logarithmically coded numbers. No multiplications would be needed with the vector quantization method, and no exponential functions would be needed when using the normal distribution.

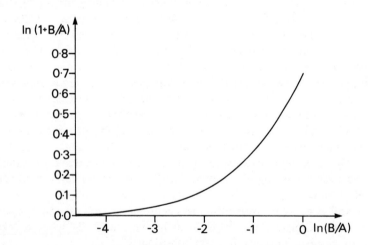

Fig. 8.3　Shape of the function required in a look-up table for efficient calculation of $\ln(A+B)$, given $\ln(A)$ and $\ln(B)$.

8.12 CONSEQUENCES OF INSUFFICIENT TRAINING DATA (PART 2)

In section 8.7 and 8.8 we considered ways of estimating model parameters with only moderate amounts of training data. Of the two methods described, modelling the features by a multi-variate normal distribution has generally been found more effective with limited training, so this method will be assumed in this section.

If a word recognizer is intended to be used with a particular speaker, it is usual for the speaker to previously 'train' the recognizer by speaking several examples of all the permitted words. Unfortunately, even for such a moderate amount of training, the process becomes extremely tedious for the speaker unless the vocabulary is very small. The computation for the parameter estimation can also take a very long time, particularly if the vocabulary is fairly large, so there is a great incentive to keep the number of training examples for each word as small as possible.

Provided the training procedure is such as to ensure that the individual training words cover a fair range of the different pronunciations that will occur in operational use, useful modelling of the variability of most of the features can be achieved even with only four or five examples of each word. However, with such a small number it is highly likely that a few of the features will, by chance, have much less than their expected variation, and so will give very small variances in the p.d.f.s for the assumed normal distribution. The effect will be to make many of the words match their models very badly for a high proportion of the time, and so cause recognition errors.

If practical considerations preclude the use of a large number of examples to form the word models, it is safest also to take into account any *a priori* knowledge we have about likely variance of features. For example, with a filter-bank analyser it seems very likely that the output of a channel for a particular frame of a particular word will vary by at least 2 – 3 dB from occasion to occasion. This fact could be used as a guide to impose a minimum value for the variance of a feature if the calculated value is less than the expected minimum.

Similar problems arise in estimating transition probabilities, particularly if the number of states is approximately equal to the number of frames. *A priori* knowledge is useful for this purpose also, to prevent plausible paths through the states from being heavily penalized merely because they are not well represented in the training data.

Obviously stochastic recognizers will give better performance when given adequate training. However, if sensible account is taken of *a priori* knowledge, even with very small amounts of training data they offer a substantial improvement over pattern-matching methods that use only one example of each word.

8.13 EXTENSION OF HIDDEN MARKOV MODELS TO WORD SEQUENCES

In the same way as was done with dynamic programming in Chapter 7, it is possible to extend hidden Markov models for connected sequences of words. The states of this higher-level model will then correspond to whole words, and the transition probabilities will be the probabilities of the possible word pairs in the language used with the machine.

In the case of recognition of individual words we were not interested in the state sequences as such, but only in the total likelihood of each word model emitting the observed feature vectors. When applying Markov models to connected words, however, we would require to know the most likely sequence of words, so in this case the Viterbi algorithm is appropriate.

Provided the Viterbi algorithm is used for determining likelihoods within words, the word-boundary procedure is exactly analogous to that described in section 7.10, making use of the back-pointers to determine the word sequences. However, if the total likelihood method is used (e.g. to gain the better time-modelling that is possible with a generous allocation of states) there is no unique path back from each point, and therefore back-pointers within the word cannot strictly exist. When calculating the likelihood for each state with a new input frame, it is, however, possible to identify the largest of the separate contributions to the new likelihood. The back-pointer for the largest such contribution could then be carried forward to the new frame, exactly as with the Viterbi algorithm. Although this method of determining word sequences lacks the elegance of the standard maximum-likelihood technique and is not normally used, it might still offer the time-modelling benefits of the total likelihood calculation. Other techniques for connected words are also possible.

Methods of extending hidden Markov models to deal with very large vocabularies, taking into account word-sequence probabilities in models of language, will be discussed in the next chapter.

SUMMARY
Chapter 8

The performance of pattern-matching speech recognizers is improved if they take into account the fact that some parts of words are more variable than others. One approach is to produce a stochastic model of each word. Hidden Markov models represent each word as a sequence of states, with transition probabilities between each state and its permitted successors, and probability distributions defining the expected observed features for each state. It is possible to use a recursive formula to calculate the probability that each word model will produce the observed data. The model with the highest probability is assumed to represent the correct word.

Some computation savings can be achieved by using the Viterbi dynamic programming algorithm to compute the probability of producing the data from only the most probable path through the states of the model. This probability will always be less than the true probability, but in most circumstances it is good enough to provide a useful recognition performance.

For each word model the transition probabilities and the probability distributions of the feature vectors can be found by the Baum–Welch re-estimation process, which successively refines initial guesses. The re-estimation requires many examples of each word as training data.

Vector quantization can be used to reduce the range of feature vectors, and so make it easier to get reliable statistics from limited training data. A parametric model, such as the normal distribution, can also be used to describe the feature statistics, and the re-estimation can be applied to parameters of the model.

A hidden Markov model with very few states is inadequate for choosing between words whose main difference is duration. The full benefit from providing several more states is not obtained if the Viterbi algorithm is used.

The dynamic programming method described in Chapter 7 can be shown to be equivalent to the use of a very primitive hidden Markov model.

One way of overcoming scaling problems because of very small numbers in the calculations is to represent all the numbers by their logarithms, and to use a special technique for finding the logarithm of the sum of two numbers.

Hidden Markov models can be extended to deal with word sequences, in which each state of the model represents one word, and the transition probabilities are determined by word sequence statistics of the language.

EXERCISES
Chapter 8

E8.1 What is the significance of the word 'hidden' in hidden Markov model recognizers?

E8.2 Why is it possible to avoid explicit consideration of all possible state sequences when calculating the probability of a hidden Markov model generating observed data?

E8.3 What is the essential difference between the Viterbi algorithm and the total likelihood method when calculating the probability of a word model generating observed data? What practical advantage can be gained by using the Viterbi algorithm?

E8.4 How can the form of an HMM be constrained by choice of initial parameters provided for re-estimation?

E8.5 What is the purpose of the 'vector quantization' that is sometimes used in HMM recognizers?

E8.6 What are the benefits of using normal distributions to model feature statistics in HMMs?

E8.7 Why does the Viterbi algorithm not give the full benefit that can result from a generous allocation of states?

E8.8 Give two reasons why Baum–Welch re-estimation is not suitable for determining time-scale distortion penalties in DTW recognizers.

E8.9 Describe the Kingsbury–Rayner technique for adding numbers that are only available in logarithmic form.

E8.10 Why should *a priori* speech knowledge be taken into account when training HMM recognizers?

9

SPEECH RECOGNITION FOR VERY LARGE VOCABULARIES

9.1 PROBLEMS WITH EXTENDING SMALL-VOCABULARY METHODS

The speech recognition methods described in the previous two chapters are usually used with vocabulary sizes ranging from a dozen to a few hundred words. There are many practical tasks where recognizers using these methods are already in widespread operation and for which these sizes of vocabulary are adequate. The applications are mainly for control of and data entry into machines of various sorts.

Whole word pattern-matching methods are not applicable as they stand to very large vocabularies (i.e. several thousand words or more). There are three main reasons for the vocabulary size limitation:

1 The amount of memory and computation required to store and compare all the patterns (or word models) becomes excessive. Although with present technology this limitation is still important, it is becoming less serious with each year of technological development.
2 Although required in the enrolment process, it is very inconvenient for the intended users to speak all the permitted words even once. To generate stochastic models, several utterances of each word would be needed. Even for a very dedicated user, the enormous time needed for enrolment would probably prevent speech recognition from being considered for several otherwise suitable applications.
3 When the number of words is large, particularly for continuous speech, variations in pronunciation of one word will often exceed the measured

differences between examples of different words. Under these circumstances recognition errors will be unavoidable.

This last limitation is the most fundamental, and there are several reasons for the variability which causes it, described below.

Example words used for training will show systematic influences from co-articulation at the beginning and end, depending on the particular phonetic environment in which they are spoken. Simple pattern matching would be disturbed by this co-articulation. A Markov model would give less weight to the variable parts in the matching process, but would not in itself take any account of the fact that the variability was systematically related to the environment.

Another serious problem is caused by the fact that chance variability in one part of a word may be greater than phonetically-caused differences between words. This effect is particularly severe for the simpler pattern-matching systems, which tend to give equal importance to equal duration events. Thus a small and irrelevant difference is articulation of a long vowel may give a greater accumulated matching error than a short-duration difference in a stop consonant that arises because the words are actually different.

Further variability of patterns to be matched arises as a result of differences of emphasis, or other effects related to pitch and timing of an utterance.

For all of the above reasons most current attempts to recognize large vocabularies have abandoned pattern matching of stored whole words and are trying other methods. The methods described in this chapter are the subject of current research, and none has solved the general problem of large-vocabulary speech recognition. A few of the more elaborate systems that have been developed are, however, capable of performing useful but restricted tasks, and the main potential applications can be split into two general classes, which are described in the next section.

9.2 SPEECH TRANSCRIPTION AND SPEECH UNDERSTANDING

As with the contrast between speech synthesis from text and synthesis from concept, there are two quite distinct sorts of application for large-vocabulary recognizers. For speech transcription, the user wishes to know exactly what the speaker said, in the form that it would normally be transcribed by an audio typist. For speech understanding, the semantic content of the message is required, and it is of no consequence if there are errors in identifying the less important words provided the meaning is not thereby changed.

Understanding systems are mostly applicable to man–machine dialogue, such as might be required for a computerized database enquiry system, or for automatic medical diagnosis by means of a question and answer session with patients. In tasks such as these, the machine would only have to work over a restricted range of subject areas, and the vocabulary might then be made much smaller than the size that is used in normal speech; a size as small as 1000 – 2000 words would be useful in many cases. If the speaker uses occasional unknown words there might be sufficient constraint on the possible meanings for the message still to be correctly interpreted.

Although for transcription one should, in principle, transcribe everything that is said, including any stuttering, hesitation noises, slips of the tongue, etc., there are few applications where this would be desirable. The human transcriber corrects most of these errors by virtue of understanding the text, but to do this successfully the vocabulary of the transcriber needs to be extremely large to give confidence that the speaking errors are not merely unknown words. For the foreseeable future, therefore, it seems that automatic speech transcription is unlikely to cope with incorrectly spoken text.

The interpretation parts of a speech understanding system require the techniques of artificial intelligence. These will include methods of parsing sentences so that the syntactic function of words can be determined. It is necessary to make a semantic analysis based on the normal meaning of the words, and also to take into account pragmatic knowledge related to the particular subject of discourse and other information already known to the system. A typical human listener uses information of these types in a very complicated way, and this use greatly increases the ability to cope with indistinctly spoken material and with utterances which require extensive inference of subject matter from previous parts of the dialogue. The most advanced current techniques for dealing with these processes are still very limited compared with human performance, but their details are outside the scope of this book.

9.3 PHONETIC FEATURES

Some of the earliest work on automatic speech recognition, in the 1950s, avoided the pattern-matching methods that are so widely used today. It seemed obvious to many of the early workers, from looking at spectrograms, for example, that the sound properties associated with different phonemes were quite characteristic, and that it should be possible, by measuring acoustic properties, to transcribe speech directly into phonemes. The techniques employed typically involved measuring such quantities as zero-crossing rate of the waveform or the rate of build-up of power. The former gives an approximate indication of the balance between high- and low-frequency power, and the latter would be useful for detecting stop consonant bursts. Not surprisingly, these early techniques were able to detect some phonetic events quite reliably, but others were much more difficult. For example, sound patterns associated with $/s/$ are fairly characteristic in having most of their power above 4 kHz and lasting at least 50 ms. For other fricative consonants, such as $/f/$, the power level is normally much less than for $/s/$.

However, the spectral distribution of power associated with these two phonemes will not be that much different except for the higher frequencies, which may not be available in a system of limited bandwidth. Unfortunately a weaker than average [s] may then not be reliably different from a stronger than average [f].

The same types of effects apply to most of the other phonemes, and the problem is made more difficult by the fact that it is often not even possible to tell how many phonemes there are in a cluster of vowels or consonants. The actual sound pattern at the end of a word like 'coughs', which is phonemically a sequence of two items, /fs/, will actually show a smooth change of properties, and there will be no clear point in time where one can say the [f] has stopped and the [s] has started. Determination of the number of phonemes is even more difficult at the junction of two words that end and start with the same phoneme, such as 'in November'.

A particular reason for the poor results of these early systems was the fact that they relied almost entirely on the intuitions of the experimenter, who generally developed *ad hoc* rules, often to a large extent influenced more by what was easy to implement with 1950s electronic technology than by what was really required. Because the primary skill for this work needed to be electronic circuit design, it was usual for the speech research workers of this period to be further handicapped by having no training in phonetics and linguistics.

Although the simple approaches of the 1950s showed extremely limited success, the same idea underlies some of the large-vocabulary recognition research of today. The differences are:

1 There is now a much better understanding of the relationship between the acoustic and the phonetic properties. This understanding is exemplified by the fact that a few highly-trained individuals can actually make a fairly accurate phonemic transcription of nonsense words using only spectrographic evidence.

2 With modern computing systems we can do much more elaborate processing than was feasible in the 1950s. It is therefore possible to implement quite complicated rules to determine the probability of particular phonemes being represented by the sound pattern at particular places in an utterance, taking into account allophonic variation expected as a result of the sound pattern on either side.

3 The greater computational power also means it is now practicable to offer several alternative analyses of a particular sound segment, with a weighing of evidence to derive estimates of the relative probabilities of the occurrence of different phonemes. It is then left to some higher level to interpret the alternative phonetic sequences to give valid words and phrases etc.

9.3.1 Expert systems

To use the phonetic feature approach, it is necessary to take into account the large number of different acoustic cues to particular minimal phonetic differences, and it is very difficult to formulate the rules for making some fine phonetic distinctions. For example, it has been claimed that there are 16 different acoustic features that can contribute to the perception of the voiced/voiceless distinction for a stop consonant when it is preceded and followed by a vowel (e.g. the distinction between /t/ and /d in 'seating' and 'seeding'). It is therefore not a trivial task merely to collect the information that relates these multiple cues to the various phonetic interpretations. A method commonly adopted for this process is to accept that some very skilful human beings can perform the interpretation task. It is then necessary to assist the human to state his/her rules explicitly and to transfer them into a machine, perhaps using some form of 'expert system'. If the human skill is independent of the properties of the speech of different talkers, these rules should then be speaker independent.

Speech recognition methods that depend primarily on capturing human knowledge to formulate rules are often referred to as **knowledge-based.**

9.3.2 Phonetic feature detection using statistical methods

Instead of using an expert system to formulate specific acoustic/phonetic rules, one can use the human knowledge in a different way. The human expert has some idea of what types of acoustic features are likely to be useful for making phonetic decisions, and can therefore specify measurement techniques that will indicate the extent to which features of these types are present. The use of a model of the peripheral auditory system (see Chapter 3) can highlight phonetically important features to some extent, but the process referred to here is more powerful because the features may be derived from complicated and time-varying functions of various durations, such as formant transitions of a particular rate. To relate the features to phonetic properties, one can prepare a large amount of phonetically labelled speech, and program a machine to analyse this speech to measure the values of the features associated with each label. The output of this analysis would not be yes/no decisions of whether or not a feature is present, but would be an indication of how much the feature is in evidence. It is thus possible to specify a probability of each phone as a function of the measurements. These data can be used as input to various interpretation procedures.

With this statistical feature approach the mathematics will be more tractable if one can assume normal distributions for each measured feature value. This assumption implies having many different allophones for each phoneme, because otherwise there would be a danger of multi-modal distributions of some features as a result of phonemically equivalent alternative pronunciations in different phonetic environments.

In the process of measuring the statistics for each allophone, the results will obviously be dependent on the speaker. Although it would in principle be possible to lump together data from a large number of speakers, this process could be very dangerous, particularly if there were significant differences of physiology or accent between them. In this situation also, the difficulty is caused by the likelihood that the distribution from multiple speakers will depart significantly from normal. Attempting to develop speaker-independent rules for each allophone is, in any case, likely to restrict performance, because it ignores the useful fact that the whole of any one utterance will come from the same speaker.

One method of reducing the computation in processing statistical features is to use a tree-structured decision process. In this method the allophones are first divided into classes that are found to have very significant differences in certain features or combinations of features. Every class is further subdivided by examining other combinations of features within the class. The class boundaries are found by analysis of the feature measurements for input with known phonetic content. Unfortunately this tree-structured decision method is likely to make errors when the evidence for the first division is very near the decision boundary. If the choice is then made the wrong way, more detailed evidence in the feature pattern in favour of a particular allophone the other side of the boundary can never correct the error.

9.4 SEGMENT LATTICE

The phonetic analysis of a speech signal needs to be represented in a way that the subsequent processing can conveniently handle. A popular way of making such a representation is to identify all points in time which the feature evidence suggests are near a phonetic segment boundary, and to attach labels between pairs of boundary points indicating which segments are possible in those periods. It would be normal also to include a number with each segment label to indicate the strength of the acoustic evidence supporting its choice. A typical fragment of a segment lattice is shown in Fig. 9.1 for the word sequence 'Let me see'.

The task of the linguistic processing is to find the best path through the whole utterance that joins the segments end to end, taking into account both the strength of the phonetic evidence and the syntactic, semantic and pragmatic constraints.

9.5 BOTTOM-UP AND TOP-DOWN PROCESSING

Even if the allophone string produced from a continuous speech input is

Time
→

/	l	e	t	m	i:	s	i:	/
l 0.8	e 0.7	p 0.6	m 0.6	e 0.5	ɪ 0.8	s 0.8	ɪ 0.8	i: 0.7
r 0.2	ɪ 0.3	t 0.3	n 0.4	i: 0.6		f 0.2	i: 0.44	
		k 0.1						

Fig. 9.1 The type of segment lattice one might expect for the phrases 'Let me see'. The phonemic transcription of the sentence is shown at the top, and the hypothesized segments are shown below. The symbol /ɪ/ represents the vowel phoneme used in the word 'sit' and /i:/ represents the vowel in 'seat'. The numbers after each segment name represent estimates of the relative likelihoods of those segments being present. With the likelihoods as shown the words spoken would not be given by the most likely segment sequence based on the acoustic evidence alone.

unambiguous and 100% accurate, the interpretation into words still depends on decisions about the word-boundary locations. In practice there will be alternative interpretations for a high proportion of the allophones, and at some places none of the alternatives will represent the correct phoneme, so there will often be substantial difficulty in determining a word sequence.

One method of interpreting a segment lattice is to start at the beginning of the sequence with the phonemes judged to be most likely, and then to test for successively increasing numbers of phonemes whether they specify a valid word of the language. As soon as a valid word is found one can start again looking for the next word etc. This operation is known as **bottom-up** processing, because it starts at the lowest linguistic level and works upwards to derive the message. A variant of this method is to start the processing with a group of phonemes for which the acoustic evidence is least ambiguous, and to work outwards from this group in both directions.

The problems with bottom-up processing arise when there is either ambiguity about word boundaries, or actual errors in the allophone recognition. When it turns out to be impossible to find a valid word, or where after an early valid word the only one which could follow it according to the acoustic evidence is ruled out because it does not conform to linguistic rules, one has to back-track and investigate the next alternative. This alternative might involve a different choice of word boundary, or perhaps a different choice for one of the allophones that was not very certain from the acoustic evidence. Bottom-up processing by itself can result in a very large amount of back-tracking, particularly when the raw material is fairly prone to errors.

An alternative to bottom-up processing is **top-down**. The method here is to postulate the most likely linguistic message, based on knowledge of the recognition task, information that has already been given, etc. This message is then converted into an allophone sequence, which is compared with the input and either accepted, if it fits sufficiently well, or otherwise rejected. If rejected, the next most likely message is tested similarly.

Top-down processing also involves trying an extensive range of possibilities, so neither method on its own is very satisfactory. It is usually better to try some combination of both methods. At the beginning of the recognition process there is not normally much indication about what the message should be from linguistic or semantic evidence, so it is better to rely mainly on the acoustic evidence to choose possible first-guess words. Once a few words have been found which fit the acoustic pattern fairly well, one can then avoid the work of bottom-up search by using those words to guide the most probable choice of the remaining items by top-down processing.

In general the balance between bottom-up and top-down will depend on how accurate the acoustic interpretation is, and how much the knowledge of the task domain constrains the messages. Bottom-up analysis is more successful when provided with better acoustic interpretation. With more linguistic constraints, it becomes practicable to reduce the work load by making earlier use of the top-down approach.

9.6 USE OF HIDDEN MARKOV MODELS FOR LARGE VOCABULARIES

Although the hidden Markov model approach for matching of whole words is not practicable for very large vocabularies, the same principles can be applied with different size units. For example, the relationship between allophones and their acoustic measurements can be represented as a statistical model, and so can the choice of allophones to represent each phoneme in a word. Similarly, the rules about likely word sequences can also be modelled in the form of transition probabilities. It is then possible to model a complete language in the form of a network of states, which represents the linguistic structure at many levels. At the lowest level a small network representing a short sequence of acoustic measurements can be regarded as one state representing an allophone. A network of allophones will form a state to represent a word. A complete sentence can then be generated just by a network of word states, or it could be considered as a sequence of larger syntactic or semantic units, each represented by a network of words describing a higher-level state in the model.

In the recognition process the linguistic content of the utterance is assumed to be given by the maximum-likelihood path through the highest level units of the model. The possibility of recognizing connected speech by this form of multi-level hidden Markov process was first pointed out by Baker (1975), in his classic work on the DRAGON system at Carnegie-Mellon University.

To be able to use a first-order hidden Markov model, it is necessary to make certain idealizing assumptions about the signal. In particular, at each level it has to be assumed that the probability of generating any event depends only on the identity of the current state, and the probability of a transition from a given state to any other state depends only on the identities of the source and destination states. Both of these probabilities are independent of the path by which the model reached its current state. It is, of course, obvious that the assumptions of the model are not really true for human speech. The properties of individual phones often depend on several surrounding phones. Word sequence probabilities are influenced by very complex factors involving the structure of complete sentences and larger units. The actual acoustic measurements for a given allophone are highly dependent on other factors, such as prosody. It has to be determined by experiment whether a sufficient performance can be achieved in spite of these limitations.

If the model represents the properties of real speech sufficiently well, it is possible to measure the probability distributions for the acoustic levels entirely by training on a sufficient quantity of phonetically labelled speech. The phonetic spelling of the words and the word sequence probabilities cannot be obtained in this way for large vocabulary systems because it is impracticable to supply enough training data. However, a pronouncing dictionary can provide standard pronunciations for each word, and then phonological rules can be applied to generate alternative allophone sequences. If however, the known phonological rules fail to provide some valid allophone sequences, the acoustic effect of allophonic variation can still be modelled and will merely manifest itself as greater variability of those allophones that are most similar to the ones that are missing.

It would be completely impracticable to provide sufficient speech data to determine the word sequence transition probabilities, but they can be estimated from any available representative large corpus of written text. However, many plausible sequences of words may never, in fact, occur even in a very large body of text, so it is necessary to give some small but finite probability to grammatically valid possibilities that are not actually found.

Although these techniques are still in the development stage, multi-level hidden Markov models have been quite successfully used for some fairly large-vocabulary systems. The use of delayed decisions is a very important basic principle of this Markov-model approach which contributes to its present level of success with some quite difficult problems.

The interpretation of a message involves evaluating the probability of the model generating the observed data along all possible paths through a network structure. Although probabilities of all valid partial paths are evaluated, effectively in parallel, no decisions are reached until all earlier parts of a path enter the same highest-level state at the same time, thus delaying decisions until all relevant evidence has been used. The path up to the confluent state will then be the maximum-likelihood path through the model up to that point, given the data.

Although there are, in general, several paths out of each state in the model, there are also several paths into each state. When the model decodes the input data, the paths through the network recombine at the same rate as new paths are formed. The computation thus increases only linearly with the length of the utterance.

9.7   THE IBM DICTATION MACHINE

One of the most ambitious current systems using Markov techniques is the **Tangora** system from IBM's Thomas J. Watson Research Center (Jelinek, 1985, contains an excellent overview of the system as it was at the time). Tangora is a demonstration system for automatic dictation of office correspondence, implemented on a personal computer supplemented by extra signal processing modules. One version is capable of handling a vocabulary of 20 000 English words with fairly high accuracy, and with provision for easy correction of errors observed by the operator. On a practical dictation task many of the errors will arise merely because 20 000 words will not cover all the words people actually use. To ease this problem, provision has been made for the user to add extra words to the vocabulary appropriate for particular types of text.

The Tangora system has to be trained by each user, and the training is done be analysing 20 minutes of speech from a text known to the machine. This text is sufficiently large to ensure that each possible phoneme should occur many times in a variety of phonetic environments. The acoustic analysis uses an auditory model to provide a 20-dimensional acoustic feature vector every 10 ms, which gives implicit emphasis to phonetically important features in the speech. However, the process of phonetic feature detection is merely the result of training the Markov models for all possible phones, and does not directly incorporate the phonetic knowledge of human experts.

The language model is derived from the statistics of three-word sequences taken from 27 million words of office correspondence. Although this seems a large number, there will be a very high proportion of valid sequences of the less common words that will not occur at all. In fact, 27 million allows just one occurrence of each possible triplet in a vocabulary of only 300 words. The IBM team have devoted a significant part of their work to devising techniques for deriving their language model from such sparse data.

The use of word triplet statistics is not consistent with the usual first-order Markov assumption. If, however, the maximum-likelihood algorithm (see sections 8.4 and 8.13) is used to derive the path leading to each word state, the identity of the previous word on that path will also be known. It is therefore possible to use word triplet probabilities to determine the transition probabilities for all following words, taking into account the most likely preceding word.

In spite of the impressive performance of the Tangora system, it still falls far short of what an audio typist can do with ease, in terms of accuracy and versatility. In particular, besides the need for training with each speaker, it has not been possible to achieve a satisfactory performance without requiring a short silence to separate every pair of words. Although the algorithms used in Tangora do not in principle require gaps between the words, there are two important benefits from providing them. First, it makes it extremely unlikely that the machine will find acoustically plausible but incorrect words that straddle the boundaries of the actual words spoken. Second, it reduces the co-articulation across word boundaries and so improves the consistency of the patterns for each word.

9.8 ALLOWING FOR CO-ARTICULATION

Although expert system rules for analysis of phonetic features can include allowance for co-articulation by having explict rules for each phonetic environment, it is a major task to formulate all the rules sufficiently accurately. With first-order Markov models for allophones, co-articulation cannot be modelled properly unless enough allophones can be included to allow for all the various forms that occur for each phoneme. It is clearly sub-optimal merely to include the allophonic variation in the statistics of the states of a phone model because such variation is systematically related to the identities of neighbouring phones.

It is possible to make some allowance for co-articulation between adjacent phones by using a diphone method, by direct analogy with the diphone synthesis described in Chapter 5. With this method it is necessary to make the set of diphones correspond to the speech of the individual talker, and then to find the best way of describing the speech as a sequence of diphones, either by dynamic programming or the HMM technique. If the HMM method is used it is possible to include transition probability information for the higher levels exactly as for the systems with single-phone models. In the case of diphones one would, of course, have the additional constraint that transitions from any diphone are only possible to other diphones that match at the join, so the branching factor at each junction will be roughly equal to the square root of the number of diphones provided.

Although some laboratories have tried using diphone units for experiments in automatic speech recognition, many of the limitations of modelling speech with diphones that were mentioned in Chapter 5 are equally applicable for recognition. One particular recognition problem is that of irrelevant variation, mentioned in section 9.1 in connection with whole-word matching. Let us assume that we are trying to recognize an input word 'net', which might be confused with 'met'. These two words are acoustically very similar, although there is usually a small but consistent difference between the sound patterns for /n/ and /m/ for a given speaker. However, there will also be substantial but irrelevant variations between different examples of the vowel

/e/. It is therefore quite likely that there will sometimes be a better match of the input /ne/ to the /me/ diphone than to the /ne/ diphone, merely because of a better match to the vowel.

9.9 USING SYNTHESIS BY RULE AS A MODEL FOR SPEECH RECOGNITION

One way of modelling co-articulation between phones, and taking into account the effect of more phonetic environment than is possible with diphones, is to use rule synthesis for generating the speech models. This method completely removes the effects of irrelevant variation, because the only variations in the models will be those caused by substituting one phoneme for another. Even if the input speech is rather a poor match to the model, the right phoneme in any position should then usually match better than the wrong one.

With models based on synthesis the interpretation can still be done with a hierarchy of unit sizes, just as with the Markov models. It is, in principle, possible to generate models for whole words dynamically as required, incorporating the sorts of prosodic properties that are observed in the input speech being recognized. Word-boundary co-articulation is automatically provided by this method.

Very little work has yet been done to investigate the value of rule-synthesized speech in a recognition system. So far, speech generated by rule has not been good enough to provide a close acoustic match to natural speech, even when it has been highly intelligible. Making the distance metric more directly related to phonetic difference should help substantially. Improving the synthesis rules, and making them adapt automatically to the speech of particular talkers, would obviously be a great advantage. Some method of indicating the amount of random variation allowable at various points in an utterance is also desirable.

In spite of the formidable difficulties, there seems to be a considerable value in investigating methods based on synthesis. Many of their potential advantages also apply to medium-vocabulary systems, particularly for connected words because of the automatic word-boundary co-articulation.

SUMMARY Chapter 9

Whole word pattern matching is not suitable for very large vocabularies because of difficulty in training and because of variation in the way words are spoken on different occasions.

Small vocabularies are mostly used for machine control and data entry, but large vocabularies have application for speech transcription and for speech understanding in man–machine dialogue. Both applications benefit from knowledge of the language structure, but speech understanding also requires extensive use of artificial intelligence techniques.

Many laboratories are using phonetic feature detectors for large vocabulary recognition, with either explicit rules or statistical classification methods to determine possible phoneme sequences. Possible phonemes can then be arranged in a segment lattice, with a combination of bottom-up and top-down processing to derive likely word sequences.

An alternative approach is to use a multi-level hidden Markov model, in which the lower-level states correspond to individual allophones and the higher levels represent phonemes, words or larger syntactic or semantic units. The Markov approach has the advantage of delaying decisions until all relevant information has been used, so avoiding the back-tracking of bottom-up and top-down methods.

IBM have a demonstration dictation transcriber for isolated words that uses Markov techniques, including a language model based on the statistics of word triplet frequencies in 27 million words of office correspondence.

Diphone methods offer some improvements for modelling co-articulation. Word models generated by rule should, in due course, be able to provide for co-articulation, and will eliminate the irrelevant variation that arises when using the other methods with insufficient training data.

EXERCISES
Chapter 9

E9.1 Why is it not practicable to extend the methods described in Chapters 7 and 8 to very large vocabularies?

E9.2 Explain the different requirements and problems in speech transcription and speech understanding.

E9.3 Give examples of how human acoustic/phonetic knowledge can be used in the design of large vocabulary speech recognizers.

E9.4 Why is a dictionary specifying all permitted words essential for large vocabulary speech recognition?

E9.5 Explain the difference between bottom-up and top-down processing.

E9.6 Explain how hidden Markov models can be extended to large vocabulary recognition using a hierarchy of states

E9.7 Explain how speech synthesis by rule could be employed in large vocabulary speech recognition.

10

POSSIBLE FUTURE RESEARCH DIRECTIONS FOR SPEECH SYNTHESIS AND RECOGNITION

10.1 INTRODUCTION

Although existing performance of speech synthesizers and recognizers makes them already extremely useful for a variety of practical tasks, this performance falls far short of what is normally achieved with ease by human beings. In speech synthesis, the best current systems either produce highly intelligible speech of very good quality for a very restricted set of messages, or they can produce a wide range of messages that are significantly deficient compared with typical human speech in both intelligibility and naturalness. In recognition, even the most advanced of current machines cannot provide an accuracy that approaches what is achievable by a competent human speaker of the target language, except when the task is so constrained that the machine has very few output choices at any time.

Although the task of improving performance of speech input/output devices is not trivial, there are a number of lines of work that show considerable promise.

The first point to emphasize is that although immense complexity will be required in more powerful systems, the technology of implementation in electronic circuits is not likely to be the limiting factor. In the past the digital signal processing and other computation involved in synthesis and recognition has been the dominant factor in the cost of products and in many cases has made the advantages of using speech technology insufficient to justify the expense. This situation still applies to a large extent now, but there is every reason to assume that the continuing downward trend of electronic circuit costs will make expense less of a disadvantage in future. However, the limitations of speed in such circuits is likely to require the use of large numbers of computing devices in parallel to achieve the computational power needed for the more advanced equipments. Although parallelism is an inconvenience for the traditional algorithms that are essentially serial in their operation, there are other approaches, described in section 10.5, that intrinsically require a parallel architecture for efficient implementation.

For most research purposes, the complexity of techniques being tried in the better-equipped laboratories is not being significantly limited by the cost of hardware, but by the difficulties of assessing (for synthesis) or providing (for recognition) sufficient quantities of speech for testing new algorithms.

10.2 SPEECH SYNTHESIS

Current performance of synthesis by rule, even when a correct phonemic and prosodic specification is provided, would almost never be mistaken for a recording of human speech. The potential sources of the deficiency are in the speech production model and in the rules for controlling it. However, demonstrations made more than 10 years ago (Holmes, 1973) showed for a few sentences that it was possible to make synthetic utterances with a parallel-formant synthesizer which were almost indistinguishable perceptually from recordings of the natural utterances which they were copying. There is thus a strong implication that formant synthesizers are already available which are good enough for almost perfect synthesis by rule, and that the limitations are entirely in the rules for converting the phonemic/prosodic description into control signals for the synthesizer.

The most advanced current rules for this lower level of the speech synthesis process have provision for the main co-articulation between consecutive phonemes, and they also have some allophonic substitution rules. However, they do not normally provide for sufficient allophonic variation, in particular when allophonic differences are caused by articulatory influences a few phonemes away from the phone being synthesized.

Because phonetic rules only need to operate slowly, there is no difficulty in implementing much more complicated rules in a simple microprocessor. The trouble is that we do not yet know how to specify these rules in computationally useful form. There is a very large amount of work needed by suitably skilled experimental phoneticians to investigate all the possible circumstances in which allophonic variation is required, and then to devise suitable rules to describe what happens. Given the right tools and enough people, most of the problems at this level for any chosen language should be soluble within a very few years. It would, however, in the long term probably be more profitable to use research effort to devise methods of inferring the rules automatically from phonemically transcribed natural speech, as suggested in Chapter 6. If these techniques were developed they could be applied to any language or dialect, given enough labelled speech data to train the system.

Similar arguments to those given above apply to the problems of determining timing, intensity and pitch rules. Rules of these types are needed to supply additional information with the phonemic description, to indicate the type of stress and intonation required. It is not yet clear whether the process of adjusting such rules automatically is likely to be more or less difficult than for the phonetic level.

It is the higher levels of synthesis by rule that seem to present the most difficult challenge. Conversion of arbitrary text into a really good phonemic and prosodic description must require at least some understanding of the meaning. If the input to a synthesis system is not text but some coded form of the desired underlying concepts, the problem of conversion from concept to the phonemic and prosodic specification seems just as daunting. However, there are already some important synthesis applications which could be classified as 'synthesis from concept' which are within reach of solution. For example, database enquiry systems often have to provide the user with information which is stored in a coded form that is not conventional text (e.g. train time-tables), but the conversion into a suitable specification for speaking is not too difficult in this case because of the restricted range of information that is normally offered by such systems. The more general problem of converting arbitrary concepts into speech is much more difficult, but the difficulties are generally regarded as problems of artificial intelligence, not speech technology. Most language processing work in artificial intelligence has so far only considered textual forms of language: although the achievements in this field are impressive, they are still very inadequate compared with what will be needed to make a significant difference to speech synthesis. Complete emulation of human performance is still many years away.

10.3 AUTOMATIC SPEECH RECOGNITION

The pattern-matching approaches to automatic speech recognition explained in Chapters 7 and 8, and the large-vocabulary methods described in Chapter 9, all have serious limitations.

These techniques also have some very desirable properties. The pattern-matching approach applied to continuous recognition with the one-pass algorithm explained in section 7.11 is in some ways similar to the HMM large-vocabulary method described in Chapter 9. Neither of them outputs any recognition result except where the partial trace-back through possible word sequences coalesces into a single path. This coalescence can cause the identities of a whole sequence of words to be determined simultaneously, and in fact the implied decision about the phonemic content of an early word in the sequence can be changed as a result of evidence for a later word.

Consider the phrase 'recognize speech'. When said casually this pair of words would be acoustically quite similar to 'wreck a nice beach'. However, there might be sufficient evidence in the sound of the /zs/ phoneme sequence at the boundary between the two words to make it very probable that there really were two fricative phonemes together, and, if so, the rules of English phonology would then indicate that there must be a syllable boundary between them, which would make 'beach' impossible. This evidence for the final word would then give support to the hypothesis that the first part of the phrase might be 'recognize', and so lead to the conclusion that there was probably a /g/ phoneme before the /n/, which would not have been present in the other phrase.

Besides the effect on word boundaries, there is another way in which later words can affect the decisions about earlier words. Assume that an early word is acoustically ambiguous between two possibilities. If linguistic knowledge (such as word sequence rules) indicates that a later word for which there is strong acoustic evidence could not follow one of the two early candidates, the overall decision on the utterance will be biased strongly against that word.

It can thus be seen that for each stretch of speech these one-pass continuous recognition algorithms make a single decision about the word sequence as soon as they can reliably do so, after weighing all the evidence, acoustic and linguistic, that they have available. Provided no significant information has been lost in the acoustic analysis, they make this decision without prematurely discarding any relevant information. Experiments with human speech perception (e.g. Marslen-Wilson, 1980) strongly suggest that human speech recognition behaves in a similar way.

Chapter 9 also discussed knowledge-based methods for interpreting acoustic features. In this case phonetic feature detectors can be designed that are significantly more complicated that those discovered implicitly by training typical hidden Markov models for phonemes. However, it is quite difficult with knowledge-based methods to quantify either the acoustic measurements themselves or their reliability, whereas the stochastic methods are well able to perform both of these processes within the limitations of the model structure and the available training data.

At present the **data-driven** statistical methods seem to give better per-formance than **knowledge-based** methods on most speech recognition tasks, although we know that as presently formulated they ignore much of the information in the acoustic signal that we know is important in human speech recognition. There is thus a strong implication that we ought to advance the state of the art by combining the best aspects of both methods. In principle the ability to learn by example that is characteristic of the data-driven approach could be extended to learn much more complicated phonetic features. All that is needed is to give the models a rich enough structure and then present a sufficient quantity of labelled training data. I believe that this method is not likely to work in practice for any feasible type of model and amount of training, unless we use our knowledge of the particular types of feature that are phonetically important when choosing the structure of the models. We could thus design models to cope only with the sort of features that our knowledge leads us to believe might be cues for phonetic distinctions. If model structures of these types can be specified first, using human knowledge, it will obviate the need for the learning process to discover the types of feature, in addition to their statistics for each possible allophone. The resultant reduction in training time and in the necessary amount of training data will almost certainly be essential for any practical system.

It may clarify the above point to illustrate it by an extreme example. It is well known that the short-term spectrum of speech is the raw material that is used in human speech recognition, and that certain types of phase distortion are imperceptible. These facts are a direct consequence of the filtering operation in the ear. However, the detailed waveform of the speech contains all the information, and one should therefore in principle be able to specify a stochastic model of sufficient complexity to generate waveforms directly using the time-varying correlation between combinations of sample ordinates at various delays. If a model of the right structure is trained with sufficient speech, it would presumably eventually learn the correlations that are a direct result of the peaky spectrum caused by the formants, but unless these properties had been learnt there would be no hope of the system acquiring any elaborate phonetic knowledge. The structure of a stochastic model that generated waveforms in this way would be vastly more complicated than one whose output was spectral features, and it would have many more degrees of freedom. This fact, in turn, implies the need for more training data and training time, as well as the need for much more computation to use the model after it has been trained.

10.4 THE RELATIONSHIP BETWEEN SYNTHESIS AND RECOGNITION

Most speech research groups have for many years tended to specialize in one particular facet of speech processing, and it has been fairly unusual for the same research workers to be involved in both speech synthesis and recognition. In the past the actual techniques that have been used in the two areas have seemed to be almost completely unrelated. Yet it can be seen from the discussion in this volume that for real advancement in both of these subjects the predominant need is for knowledge about the structure of speech, and its relationship to the underlying linguistic content of utterances.

The stochastic modelling techniques that are vital to the most powerful current recognition techniques are obviously relevant to finding properties of speech that should be produced in synthesis, and knowledge of the phonetic features that are found necessary for good synthesis can equally be applied to phonetically relevant analysis for recognition.

At the linguistic and semantic levels also, artificial intelligence methods will need to use information about the current speech communication task if human performance is to be approached. In particular, knowlege about the subject matter is extremely important for producing and interpreting utterances in man–machine dialogue, and must include the effect of previous utterances on the expectations of what will follow. The processes that will be needed to interpret the phonetic and prosodic properties of speech signals as text or concepts will have their counterparts in going from text or concept into speech, and both apsects should be taken into account in dialogue design.

For the above reasons I predict that the most significant progress in the more advanced forms of speech synthesis and recognition will in future come from research teams with a strong interest in both problems.

10.5 PARALLEL DISTRIBUTED PROCESSING

10.5.1 The human brain

A prominent theme throughout this book has been the importance of emulating human performance, and a large part of this requirement applies particularly to the cognitive processes. It is thus worth considering whether such emulation can be achieved by actually modelling the type of mechanism in the human central nervous system.

Although there is as yet very inadequate knowledge of the functioning of the brain, there is now quite a lot of knowledge about its most basic components – the individual nerve cells. The nerve cell or **neuron** is an electro-chemical device with a long output fibre, the **axon**, and a large number of shorter input fibres, the **dendrites**. When it receives sufficient stimulation from its dendrites it will **fire**, and will cause a small voltage pulse to travel along its axon by a progressive electro-chemical reaction. The speed of pulse along an axon is normally less than 100 m/s, and is thus many orders of magnitude below the speed of electric pulses in wires. After a neuron has fired it will become inactive for a period of a millisecond or so, during which it is not sensitive to further stimulation. The magnitude and form of the response pulse that is transmitted along the axon is independent of the size of the stimulus which caused it. The only possible variable in a neuron's output is the time of firing, and the short-term average rate of firing is a useful measure of general activity in a neuron. The quiescent period after firing imposes a maximum firing rate, and after each firing the threshold of stimulation needed to fire the neuron again gradually reduces. In fact most neurons will fire spontaneously at a low rate even in the absence of stimulation.

The axons pass in proximity to the input dendrites of other neurons, and the coupling from a pulse in the axon from one neuron will stimulate the tendency to fire in the others. These neural junctions are known as **synapses**.

The strengths of couplings at synapses vary considerably, both from one synapse to another and over time as a result of brain development and learning. Although the firing rates of individual neurons are quite low, the precise times of firing could be highly significant in their effects at the synapses: if several synapses are stimulated simultaneously there is a much higher probability of firing in the associated neuron.

Because of the involvement of electro-chemical processes, there is a large disparity (in excess of 10000:1) between the maximum speed of operation of nerve cells and modern electronic circuits. However, this speed disadvantage is compensated for by having enormous numbers of neurons continually operating in parallel. It is estimated that the number of neurons in the human brain is at least 10^{10}, and the number of effective synapses is at least 1000 times greater.

Although the above facts do not explain how the brain performs its cognitive functions, they do give some indication of the possible processes involved.

First, the individual neurons are extremely limited in what they can do. If stimulated enough they will fire, and if not they produce no response. They do not in themselves have any memory of their previous actions. There are two possible mechanisms available for memory in the brain. Long term memory can exist only in the nature of the synaptic couplings between neurons. These couplings are partly innate, and the innate features must contain the information for all instinctive reactions. Other synapses develop over time, and changes in the strengths of synaptic couplings seem to provide the only feasible mechanism for long-term memory of learnt behaviour. Short-term memory could be achieved by continually re-circulating data, where one group of neurons stimulates the firing of another group, which in turn stimulates the first group again after the transmission delay through their axons.

A very obvious way in which operation of the brain differs from the operation of normal computers is the degree of parallel processing. There is a tendency in modern high-power computing systems to include parallel operation, but even in these machines the method is merely to divide the task into parts which can be largely done separately, and to process data serially in each part. In the brain, by contrast, all parts are working together, with a continuous high degree of inter-communication between them.

10.5.2 Connectionist models

The nature and properties of the brain have inspired many research groups to investigate whether cognitive processes could be achieved in electronic or computational models that have many of the known neural properties. The most obvious requirement for such a model is to include large numbers of inter-connections between units, whose coupling weights can be modified by 'learning'. Another important feature is to make the response of the units a non-linear function of the combined input stimulation, by analogy with the firing threshold of neurons.

In most groups working in this area the aim has not been to copy the precise action of the neural mechanism. In view of the number of neurons in the brain and the impracticability of discovering the coupling weights of the synapses, accurate achievement of any cognitive operations in this way would seem unattainable. What researchers are trying to do is to generate functional models of various cognitive processes, using knowledge of neurophysiology merely as a guide to what types of operation might be plausible. The two most important features of neural processes are that the units are working in parallel, and that each operation is distributed between many such units. These methods have therefore become generally known as **parallel distributed processing** (PDP). Making acknowledgement to the vital role of the numerous connection weights between units, models of cognitive processes of this type are sometimes also known as **connectionist models**.

10.5.3   Important properties of PDP models

A PDP system must have input units, which provide the connections through which knowledge is put into the system. For sensory pattern processing such units are given signals corresponding to the response of auditory or visual sensors, but for other types of knowledge processing they could be given other suitably coded forms of information. There must also be output units, through which the response of the system is made externally available. For any practical system it is necessary to have a means for the network to learn its required behaviour by adjusting the weights of the many inter-connections. The learning is achieved by supplying example patterns to the input units in conjunction with the patterns desired from the output units in response to these inputs. A learning algorithm is used to modify the weights of the connections in a direction that makes the model make a closer approximation to the desired output.

One of the earlier PDP systems was the **perceptron** (Rosenblatt, 1962). Although the basic design of the perceptron made it a PDP device, it only had a single layer of units between input and output connections. In spite of early enthusiasm for the capabilities of perceptrons, it was shown by Minsky and Papert (1969) that this single-layer topological structure seriously limited the type of computation that it could perform. An essential feature of the more advanced present-day PDP systems is that they require 'hidden' units, not connected to input or output. Incidentally, it is apparent from our knowledge of the structure of the brain, where the input and output pathways are quite specific (e.g. the optic and auditory nerves, and various motor nerves controlling our muscles), that a high proportion of brain cells are not connected directly to either input or output nerves. Although the learning rule for the perceptron was fairly straightforward, it is only comparatively recently that satisfactory rules have been developed for modifying the connection weights of hidden units.

There are now many different types of PDP models far more advanced than the perceptron, and they are being studied by a number of researchers. Two of the most prominent groups are located in the University of California at San Diego and in Carnegie-Mellon University, Pittsburg.

A pattern-processing problem that seems well suited to PDP methods is visual pattern recognition, and techniques for this task are being widely studied. A popular structure for the purpose is similar in many ways to Rosenblatt's peceptron, except that it includes one or more layers of hidden units. The term **multi-layer perceptron** is often used to describe it.

Another type of PDP machine has the binary state of each of its units specified by a probabilistic function of the states of the units it is connected to. The equations governing the operation of this machine are closely analogous to those of statistical thermodynamics, and the relevance of the Boltzmann distribution has caused the name **Boltzmann machine** to be used. The probabilistic function controlling the states has a parameter called 'temperature', that determines how much randomness there is in the function. As the temperature approaches zero, each unit becomes more like a simple threshold device whose output state (on or off) just depends on the linear sum of its many inputs. It is possible to define a cost function associated with the global state of the entire network, which is called 'energy'. The network tends to settle into a low-energy state, in a way which optimally satisfies the constraints imposed by the combination of the inputs and the inter-connections between units. At low temperatures the global energy state will be quite stable, but the network could be stuck in a local minimum. At higher temperatures the random disturbance to the settling process will be sufficient to prevent poor local minima from being stable, but no final optimum state will be achieved. By letting the system settle while the temperature is gradually lowered, one can ensure that the final state is very close to the one that optimally satisfies all the constraints of the system. The analogy with thermal systems makes it appropriate to describe this form of constraint satisfaction as **optimization by simulated annealing**.

In contrast to most signal-processing algorithms, it is characteristic of PDP systems generally that they do not have any central control of their information flow. All parts carry on with their own allotted functions autonomously, while continually communicating with other parts. The mutual constraints on behaviour of the units, imposed by their inter-connections and the external inputs, cause a complete system to settle into a state that eventually provides results on the output units. These results will be the final consequence of attempting to satisfy the numerous constraints associated with the problem on hand. For most processes simulating human perception, none of these constraints will be mandatory. For example, a human listener can be quite confident of the identity of a word in the middle of a long sentence even when, as a result of careless articulation, the cues for one of the phonemes in the middle of that word are completely absent. A properly trained PDP machine should produce the same result if all possible alternative interpretations cause more serious inconsistencies, whereas a traditional knowledge-based feature system would have rejected the mispronounced word.

10.5.4 PDP in speech processing

Elman and McClelland (1985) of the San Diego group are strong advocates of the use of PDP for speech processing, and they have argued cogently that more traditional approaches are inherently incapable of providing a general solution to the automatic speech-recognition problem. They have already demonstrated that their TRACE model is very successful at learning many of the inter-relationships between phonetic features and phonemes. Several other groups are also taking an interest, using Boltzmann machines, multi-layer perceptions or other PDP structures.

One of the main difficulties for workers on PDP systems so far has been that they do not yet have sufficiently powerful parallel hardware to test the ideas easily. In nearly every case the research is being done by simulation using a conventional von Neumann computer architecture. This limitation has meant that learning algorithms have usually been tested on systems with no more than about a thousand units, and there have often been fewer. Although such experiments have revealed a lot about the types of properties of the various PDP networks, they have been inadequate to test their potential for the more difficult problems that other pattern-processing methods are unable to cope with.

In comparison with the hidden Markov models discussed in Chapter 9, PDP methods have the advantage that they can learn much more general types of structure, which can implement very complicated non-linear conditional rules. By varying connection weights they can also modify whatever structure they are provided with initially. In principle, therefore, these systems have the power to do most if not all of the operations involved in recognizing and interpreting speech. However, to achieve their full potential they will almost certainly need orders of magnitude more units than have been provided in any of the simulations so far. When these larger numbers of units are provided the learning problems will be immense. It seems almost certain that a large part of the human ability to do linguistic processing arises because of the innate neural connections in our brains, and actual linguistic competence then follows as a result of many years of training during which children are almost continually using language for everyday communication. Acquiring both the innate and learnt connectivity patterns seems to be a task that will not be solved in machines for many years. It seems likely that PDP applications will be more useful for speech processing in the shorter term for deriving complex rules needed for parts of the problem, in association with systems that include much of the knowledge base that experts in the subject already have.

As capabilities develop, the potential eventual gains by using PDP are such that it seems well worth allotting significant research effort to the subject now, even if the full advantages are not attainable for many years.

SUMMARY
Chapter 10

Current performance of speech synthesis and recognition machines is poor in comparison with that of humans, but the difficulty is not in the computational power achievable with electronic technology. There is, however, great difficulty in providing and analysing sufficient data to acquire the necessary speech knowledge.

Functional models of the vocal system using parallel-formant synthesis are already adequate for synthesis of excellent quality speech, but speech synthesis by rule is limited by lack of knowledge about the necessary rules.

Automatic adjustment of acoustic–phonetic rules using phonetically labelled natural speech appears to offer potential for rule development, including extension to new languages or dialects.

The most difficult synthesis problems are in making the style of speech appropriate for the intended meaning. Development of artificial intelligence techniques will be necessary.

Medium-term improvements to automatic speech recognition should be achieved by combining the best aspects of data-driven and knowledge-based methods. It is particularly important to delay decisions until there is sufficient evidence, so as to avoid back-tracking or discarding information too early.

Advanced systems both for synthesis and for recognition need the same speech knowledge, and there is considerable advantage for the two applications to be studied together.

Interest has recently developed in systems involving parallel distributed processing (PDP) to emulate various cognitive functions in ways that have some similarity to operations in the human brain. A few groups are already investigating these methods for speech processing.

If they can be given enough processing elements and sufficient training, PDP seems to have long-term potential for very powerful processing at many levels simultaneously. In the meantime the learning abilities of PDP systems might make them suitable for discovering rules of operation for more limited problems, where previous methods have not been successful because sufficient speech knowledge has not been available in usable form.

EXERCISES
Chapter 10

E10.1 Why will automatic understanding of messages be necessary for really high peformance in speech synthesis and recognition in the future?

E10.2 Mention some of the reasons why it will be extremely difficult to emulate human speech recognition performance using neural (PDP) models.

11

FURTHER READING

The subject of speech recognition and synthesis is so large that a book of this size could not hope to provide more than an overview. Most of the material presented here has made great use of published material from various sources. Although there are significant textbooks available, most of the more recent developments are covered only in specialist research papers or even in conference proceedings. This chapter aims to give sufficient information to enable the reader to trace all the important material needed for more specialized study on any of the facets of speech processing presented here.

These days nearly all speech processing is digital. One of the most important textbooks on digital processing of speech is Rabiner and Schafer (1978), but even in its early chapters this book requires the reader to be really at home with mathematical notation and manipulation. For the less mathematically minded, Witten (1982) provides a much easier introduction, though it is less comprehensive than Rabiner and Schafer.

Flanagan (1972) is a classic textbook covering a wide range of aspects of speech including quite a lot of acoustic theory. Because of recent developments, particularly in speech recognition, it is now rather dated, but it includes a very comprehensive bibliography to much of the earlier work.

Another book that includes a lot of introductory material but is also very specialized in selective areas is Fallside and Woods (1985). It contains a collection of papers by various authors, and is based on a short course run at the University of Cambridge in 1983.

There are many books of collected research papers which contain some of the significant original publications in various subject areas. Among the most important are Flanagan and Rabiner (1972), Dixon and Martin (1979) and Schafer and Markel (1979).

For those wishing to keep up with the latest developments in speech synthesis and recognition there are a few journals and regular conferences that contain nearly all the most important material. The *IEEE Transactions* on *Acoustics, Speech and Signal Processing* (monthly) is a popular location for some of the more significant papers, but only about 15% of its recent papers have been on speech subjects. The *Journal of the Acoustical Society of America* has a similar status and proportion of speech papers, but specializes in those with a more acoustical bias, including psycho-acoustics and physiological acoustics. Although these two journals have contributors from many countries, they tend to attract mostly American authors.

Speech Communication (North Holland, quarterly) is a fairly new journal devoted entirely to speech and covers all aspects. Most of its contributions so far have been from European sources. *Computer Speech and Language* (Academic Press, quarterly) is a very new journal, for which it is not yet possible to predict the scope. It is intended to be more computer-oriented than *Speech Communication*, and will include papers on language processing that do not necessarily involve speech. There are many other journals specializing in such subjects as linguistics, psychology, etc. which contain some papers on speech. They can most easily be found by studying the reference lists given in other papers on relevant subjects.

Undoubtedly the most important single annual conference covering speech processing is the IEEE International Conference on Acoustics, Speech and Signal Processing (ICASSP), usually held in the USA but occasionally in other countries. Only about 25% of its contributions are on speech, but the total size of the conference is such that there are normally at least two parallel speech sessions running throughout a four-day period, providing roughly 100 – 150 speech papers for the proceedings. Although there is quite a high proportion of less significant work, many of the most notable new achievements in speech processing are first presented at ICASSP, and the ICASSP reference is often the only published source of such work for several years.

The twice-yearly meetings of the Acoustical Society of America are another regular series of conferences. These meetings cover the same subject areas as the Society's Journal, but unfortunately the papers are only published in short abstract form, and so have little value for reference purposes. Many new research results first get published at other conferences, but it is difficult to give any general guidance because these conferences are mostly either irregular or are only run every three or four years.

As a guide to future work, as well as giving assistance in tracing past work, it is useful to search the literature for other papers by the authors mentioned in this chapter, gradually increasing one's knowledge of significant people and research groups by adding names of regular co-authors and other workers from the same laboratories.

CHAPTER 1

Although written for a completely different purpose (for teaching British

English as a foreign language), Roach (1983) provides a very readable introduction to phonetics and phonology, illustrated with examples from the 'Received Pronunciation' variety of English. O'Connor (1973) is a more general book on phonetics, and contains a useful bibliography on phonetics and linguistics.

CHAPTER 2

Fant (1960) is an important book on the acoustic theory of speech production, and Chapters 2 and 3 of Flanagan (1972) provide a general view of the mechanism of speech production and its mathematical modelling. Linggard (1985) contains an excellent chapter on the early history of acoustic models of speech production, besides dealing with many other aspects of synthesis, largely from a signal processing point of view.

Ishizaka and Flanagan (1972) and Titze (1973, 1974) describe mathematical models of the vocal folds. Holmes (1973, 1976) comments on the effects of the voiced excitation waveform in speech generation.

Flanagan et al. (1975) describe a computer model for articulatory synthesis. Klatt (1980) contains a description of a widely-used cascade/parallel formant synthesizer. Holmes (1983) presents arguments in favour of parallel formant generators for practical synthesis.

CHAPTER 3

Chapter 4 of Flanagan (1972) covers much of the acoustic aspects of hearing in fair detail. Moore (1982) is an excellent introduction to the psychology of hearing, and also includes material on auditory physiology and the physics of sound. Some innovative work on functional auditory models is given by Lyon (1982), Lyon and Dyer (1986), Seneff (1984, 1986) and Hunt and Lefèbvre (1986, 1987), all in various ICASSP proceedings.

CHAPTER 4

There are a number of useful review papers on speech coding, such as Flanagan et al. (1979) and Holmes (1982). These papers contain numerous references to earlier work on various types of coder. Markel and Gray (1976) is a complete book on linear predictive coding, including listings of computer code for some of the algorithms. More recent techniques, such as multi-pulse LPC and CELP, are given by Atal and Remde (1982), Atal (1986) and numerous other papers in more recent ICASSP proceedings. The CCITT backwards-adaptive predictor (usually called ADPCM) is described in Nishitani et al. (1985). Hess (1983) has produced a very comprehensive review of methods for measuring fundamental frequency in speech, such as are needed in vocoders. This book is outstanding in its bibliography, which spreads some way beyond its particular specialist topic.

CHAPTER 5

A typical waveform word concatenation system is described in Trupp (1970) and a formant-coded technique appears in Rabiner *et al.* (1971). Harris (1953) wrote an early paper dealing with concatenation of sub-word units (as sections of waveform). One of the earliest diphone methods, using formant coding, was described by Estes *et al.* (1964). Olive (1977) described a method using LPC coded dyads and Browman (1980) used demi-syllables.

CHAPTER 6

Klatt (1987) is a comprehensive review of methods for conversion of text to speech for English, including an extensive bibliography. The following are a small proportion of the significant publications in particular areas. Liberman *et al.* (1959) is an important early paper on acoustic/phonetic rules. Holmes *et al.* (1964) contains the first complete description of computer-implemented formant synthesis rules for all the phonemes of a language. Pierrehumbert (1981) has done some useful work on synthesizing English intonation. Allen (1987) describes MITalk, a complete text-to-speech system for American English. Young and Fallside (1979) is one of the earlier publications on synthesis from concept.

CHAPTER 7

A big improvement in whole-word pattern matching came when dynamic programming was first applied to the time-alignment problem. Vintsyuk (1968, 1971) and Velichko and Zagoruyko (1970), all from the Soviet Union, published some of the earliest work in this area. Sakoe (1979) and Bridle (1983) represent more recent work on connected word recognition. Itakura (1975) presented a linear prediction pattern-matching distance metric that has been widely used.

CHAPTER 8

This chapter requires some understanding of statistics and probability theory. There are many introductory textbooks, of which a suitable one is Bulmer (1979). The theory on which hidden Markov models are based has been discussed in a number of papers with Baum as one of the authors. An example is Baum (1972), but this paper requires the reader to have a high degree of mathematical ability. Several of the papers describing HMM methods for limited vocabulary recognition of words have come from AT&T Bell Laboratories, such as Levinson *et al.* (1983). Liporace (1982) has published a mathematical treatment of the modelling of multi-variate continuous distributions. Bourard *et al.* (1985) are the authors of a tutorial paper describing both the HMM method and dynamic programming for connected word recognition. There are many more recent papers on various aspects of stochastic recognizers in ICASSP proceedings and elsewhere.

CHAPTER 9

A general discussion of the principles of hidden Markov models as applied to large-vocabulary recognition is found in Baker (1975). The particular application to a dictating machine is described by Jelinek (1985). Knowledge-based methods are treated by De Mori and Probst (1985). A typical approach to the detection of phonetic features is given by Cole *et al.* (1986).

CHAPTER 10

It is more difficult to give references for this chapter because it is looking to the future. Some predictions are contained in Flanagan (1984) and Holmes (1984). There are some useful results about human speech recognition which are relevant to future technology in Marslen-Wilson (1980). For a very comprehensive treatment of PDP methods there is a recent pair of books edited by Rumelhart and McClelland (1986). Elman and McClelland (1985) describe the operation of their TRACE speech recognition system that uses PDP.

REFERENCES

Allen, J. (1987). *From Text to Speech: the MITalk System.* Cambridge University Press, Cambridge, England.

Atal, B. S. (1986). High-quality speech at low bit rates: multi-pulse and stochastically excited linear predictive coders. *Proc. IEEE Int. Conf. Acoustics, Speech and Signal Processing*, Tokyo, 1681–1684.

Atal, B. S. and Remde, J. R. (1982). A new model of LPC excitation for producing natural-sounding speech at low bit rates. *Proc. IEEE Int. Conf. Acoustics, Speech and Signal Processing*, Paris, 614–617.

Baker, J. K. (1975). The DRAGON system – an overview. *IEEE Trans. Acoust., Speech and Signal Process.* **ASSP-23**, 24–29.

Baum, L. E. (1972). An inequality and associated maximization technique in statistical estimation for probabilistic functions of Markov processes. *Inequalities* **III**, 1–8.

Békésy, G. von (1942). Über die Schwingungen der Schneckentrennwand beim Präparet und Ohrenmodell. *Akust. Z.* **7**, 173–186.

Bourard, H., Kamp, Y., Ney, H. and Wellekens, C. J. (1985). Speaker-dependent connected speech recognition via dynamic programming and statistical methods. In *Speech and Speaker Recognition,* Schroeder, M. R. (ed.). Karger, Basel, pp.115–148.

Bridle, J. S., Brown, M. D. and Chamberlain, R. M. (1983) Continuous connected word recognition using whole word templates. *Radio and Electronic Engineer* **53**, 167–77.

Browman, C. P. (1980). Rules for demisyllable synthesis using Lingua, a language interpreter. *Proc. IEEE Int. Conf. Acoustics, Speech and Signal Processing,* Denver, 561–564.

Bulmer, M. G. (1979). *Principles of Statistics.* Dover, New York.

Cole, R. A., Stern, R. M. and Lasry, M. J. (1986). Performing fine phonetic distinctions: templates versus features. In *Invariance and Variability in Speech Processes,* Perkell, J. S. and Klatt, D. H. (eds). Lawrence Erlbaum, Hillsdale, pp. 325–342.

De Mori, R. and Probst, D. (1985). Knowledge-based computer recognition of continuous speech. In *Speech and Speaker Recognition,* Schroeder, M. R. (ed.). Karger, Basel, pp. 53–79.

Dixon, N. R. and Martin, T. B. (eds.) (1979). *Automatic Speech and Speaker Recognition.* IEEE Press, New York.

Dudley, H. (1939). Remaking speech. *J. Acoust. Soc. Am.* **11**, 169–177.

Elman, J. L. and McClelland, J. L. (1985). An architecture for parallel processing in speech recognition: the TRACE model. In *Speech and Speaker Recognition,* Schroeder, M. R. (ed.). Karger, Basel, 6–35.

Estes, S. E., Kerby, H. R., Maxey, H. D. and Walker, R. M. (1964). Speech synthesis from stored data. *IBM J. Res. Develop.* **8**, 2–12.

Fallside F. and Woods W. A. (eds) (1985). *Computer Speech Processing.* Prentice-Hall International, London.

Fant, G. (1960). *The Acoustic Theory of Speech Production.* Mouton and Co., The Hague.

Flanagan, J. L. (1972). *Speech Analysis, Synthesis and Perception.* Springer-Verlag, Berlin.

Flanagan, J. L. (1984). Speech technology in the coming decades. In *Proceedings of the Tenth International Congress of Phonetic Sciences,* Van den Broecke, M. P. R. and Cohen, A. (eds). Foris Publications, Dordrecht, pp. 121–124.

Flanagan, J. L., Ishizaka, K. and Shipley, K. L. (1975). Synthesis of speech from a dynamic model of the vocal cords and vocal tract. *Bell Syst. Tech. J.* **54**, 485–506.

Flanagan J. L. and Rabiner, L. R. (eds) (1972). *Speech Synthesis.* Dowden, Hutchinson and Ross, Stroudsburg.

Flanagan, J. L., Schroeder, M. R., Atal, B. S., Crochiere, R. E., Jayant, N. S. and Tribolet, J. M. (1979). Speech coding. *IEEE Trans. Commun.* **COM-27**, 710–736.

Harris, C. M. (1953). A study of the building blocks of speech. *J. Acoust. Soc. Am.* **25**, 962–969.

Hess, W. (1983). *Pitch Determination of Speech Signals.* Springer-Verlag, Berlin.

Holmes, J. N. (1973). The influence of glottal waveform on the naturalness of speech from a parallel formant synthesizer. *IEEE Trans. Audio and Electroacoust.* **AU-21**, 298–305.

Holmes, J. N. (1976). Formant excitation before and after glottal closure. *Proc. IEEE Int. Conf. Acoustics, Speech and Signal Processing,* Philadelphia 39–42.

Holmes, J. N. (1982). A survey of methods of digitally encoding speech signals. *The Radio and Electronic Engineer* **52**, 267–276.

Holmes, J. N. (1983). Formant synthesizers: cascade or parallel?. *Speech Communication* **2**, 251–273.

Holmes, J. N. (1984). Speech technology in the next decades. In *Proceedings of the Tenth International Congress of Phonetic Sciences*, Van den Broecke, M. P. R. and Cohen, A. (eds). Foris Publications, Dordrecht, pp. 125–139.

Holmes, J. N., Mattingly, I. G. and Shearme, J. N. (1964). Speech synthesis by rule. *Language and Speech* 7, 127–143.

Hunt, M. J. and Lefèbvre, C. (1986). Speech recognition using a cochlear model. *Proc. IEEE Int. Conf. Acoustics, Speech and Signal Processing*, Tokyo, 1979–1982.

Hunt, M. J. and Lefèbvre, C. (1987). Speech recognition using an auditory model with pitch-synchronous analysis. *Proc. IEEE Int. Conf. Acoustics, Speech and Signal Processing*, Dallas, 813–816.

Ishizaka K. and Flanagan, J. L. (1972). Synthesis of voiced sounds from a two-mass model of the vocal cords. *Bell Syst. Tech. J.* **51**, 1233–1268.

Itakura, F. (1975). Minimum prediction residual principle applied to speech recognition. *IEEE Trans. Acoust., Speech and Signal Process.* **ASSP-23**, 67–72.

Jelinek, F. (1985). The development of an experimental discrete dictation recognizer. *Proc. IEEE* **73**, 1616–1624.

Kingsbury, N. G. and Rayner, P. J. W. (1971). Digital filtering using logarithmic arithmetic. *Electron. Lett.* **7**, 56–58.

Klatt, D. H. (1980). Software for a cascade/parallel formant synthesizer. *J. Acoust. Soc. Am.* **67**, 971–995.

Klatt, D. H. (1987). Review of text-to-speech conversion for English. *J. Acoust. Soc. Am.*, accepted for publication.

Levinson, S. E., Rabiner, L. R. and Sondhi, M. M. (1983). An introduction to the application of the theory of probabilistic functions of a Markov process to automatic speech recognition. *Bell Syst. Tech. J.* **62**, 1035–1074.

Liberman, A. M., Ingemann, F., Lisker, L., Delattre, P. and Cooper, F. S. (1959). 'Minimal rules for synthesizing speech. *J. Acoust. Soc. Am.* **31**, 1490–1499.

Lindsey, P. H. and Norman, D. A. (1972). *Human Information Processing*. Academic Press.

Linggard, R. (1985). *Electronic Synthesis of Speech*. Cambridge University Press, Cambridge, England.

Liporace, L. A. (1982). Maximum likelihood estimation for multivariate observations of Markov sources. *IEEE Trans. Information Theory* **IT-28**, 729–734.

Lyon, R. F. (1982). A computational model of filtering, detection and compression in the cochlea. *Proc. IEEE Int. Conf. Acoustics, Speech and Signal Processing*, Paris, 1282–1285.

Lyon, R. F. and Dyer, L. (1986). Experiments with a computational model of the cochlea. *Proc. IEEE Int. Conf. Acoustics, Speech and Signal Processing*, Tokyo, 1975–1978.

Markel, J. D. and Gray, A. H. Jr. (1976). *Linear Prediction of Speech*. Springer-Verlag, Berlin.

Marslen-Wilson, W. (1980). Speech understanding as a psychological process. In *Spoken Language Generation and Understanding*, Simon, J. C. (ed.), Reidel, Dordrecht.

Minsky, M. and Papert, S. (1969). *Perceptrons*. MIT Press, Cambridge, Mass.

Moore, B. C. J. (1982). *An Introduction to the Psychology of Hearing*. Academic Press, London.

Nishitani, T., Kuroda, I., Satoh, M., Katoh, T., Fukuda, R. and Aoki, Y. (1985). A CCITT standard 32 KBPS ADPCM LSI codec, *Proc. IEEE Int. Conf. Acoustics, Speech and Signal Processing*, Tampa, 1425–1428.

O'Connor, J. D. (1973). *Phonetics*. Penguin Books, Harmondsworth.

Olive, J. P. (1977). Rule synthesis of speech using dyadic units. *Proc. IEEE Int. Conf. Acoustics, Speech and Signal Processing*, Hartford, 568–570.

Pierrehumbert, J. (1981). Synthesizing intonation. *J. Acoust. Soc. Am.* **70**, 985–995.

Rabiner, L. R. and Schafer, R. W. (1978). *Digital Processing of Speech Signals.* Prentice-Hall, Englewood-Cliffs.

Rabiner, L. R., Schafer, R. W. and Flanagan, J. L. (1971). Computer synthesis of speech by concatenation of formant-coded words. *Bell Syst. Tech. J.* **50**, 1541– 1558.

Reeves, A. H. (1938). French patent 852183.

Roach, P. (1983). *English Phonetics and Phonology.* Cambridge University Press, Cambridge, England.

Robinson, D. W. and Dadson, R. S. (1956). A determination of the equal-loudness relations for pure tones. *Br. J. Appl. Phys.* **7**, 166–181.

Rose, J. E., Hind, J. E., Anderson, D. J. and Brugge, J. F. (1971). Some effects of stimulus intensity on response of auditory nerve fibers in the squirrel monkey. *J. Neurophysiol.* **34**, 685–699.

Rosenblatt, F. (1962). *Principles of Neurodynamics.* Spartan, New York.

Rumelhart, D. E. and McClelland, J. L. (1986). *Parallel Distributed Processing* (2 vols). MIT Press, Cambridge, Mass.

Sakoe, H. (1979). Two-level DP matching – a dynamic programming based pattern matching algorithm for connected word recognition. *IEEE Trans. Acoust., Speech and Signal Process.* **ASSP-27**, 588–595.

Schafer, R. W. and Markel, J. D. (eds) (1979). *Speech Analysis.* IEEE Press, New York.

Seneff, S. (1984). Pitch and spectral estimation of speech based on an auditory synchrony model. *Proc. IEEE Int. Conf. Acoustics, Speech and Signal Processing,* San Diego, paper 36.2.

Seneff, S. (1986). A computational model for the peripheral auditory system: application to speech recognition research. *Proc. IEEE Int. Conf. Acoustics, Speech and Signal Processing,* Tokyo, 1983–1986.

Titze, I. R. (1973). The human vocal cords: a mathematical model (Part 1). *Phonetica* **28**, 129–170.

Titze, I. R. (1974). The human vocal cords: a mathematical model (Part 2). *Phonetica* **29**, 1–21.

Trupp, R. D. (1970). Computer-controlled message synthesis. *Bell Lab. Record,* June/July 1970, 175–180.

Velichko, Z. M. and Zagoruyko, N. G. (1970). Automatic recognition of 200 words. *Int. J. Man-Machine Studies* **2**, 223–234.

Vintsyuk, T. K. (1968). Speech recognition by dynamic programming methods. *Kibernetika (Cybernetics)* **4**, 81–88.

Vintsyuk, T. K. (1971). Element-wise recognition of continuous speech consisting of words of a given vocabulary. *Kibernetika (Cybernetics)* **7**, 133–143.

Viterbi, A. J. (1967). Error bounds for convolutional codes and an asymptotically optimum decoding algorithm. *IEEE Trans. Information Theory* **IT-13**, 260–269.

Vogten, L. L. M. (1974). Pure tone masking; a new result from a new method. In *Facts and Models in Hearing,* Zwicker, E. and Terhardt, E. (eds). Springer-Verlag, Berlin.

Witten, I. H. (1982). *Principles of Computer Speech.* Academic Press, London.

Young, S. J. and Fallside, F. (1979). Speech synthesis from concept: a method for speech output from information systems. *J. Acoust. Soc. Am.* **66**, 685–695.

SOLUTIONS TO EXERCISES

The notes that follow give an indication of the main points that should be covered in the answers to the exercises. In many cases this indication is provided by reference to the appropriate part of the text where the information can be found.

CHAPTER 1

E1.1 Not suitable: scanning text, position control. Beneficial: data entry in hands-busy situations, or for operators without keyboard skill. Necessary: where access is only available by telephone.

E1.2 Phonetics is concerned with properties of speech sounds, phonology with their function in languages.

E1.3 See p. 8.

E1.4 See p. 4.

E1.5 See p. 5.

E1.6 See pp. 6–7.

E1.7 The enormous redundancy in the speech signal, at many levels, means that the new information needed to deduce a message is a minute fraction of that needed to specify the waveform detail. The human auditory and cognitive systems are complex enough to exploit the many forms of redundancy that are present. See pp. 8–10.

CHAPTER 2

E2.1 Voiced: harmonic, most power at low frequencies, impulsive. Voiceless: continuous spectrum, fairly even spectral distribution, continuous in time.

E2.2 Surface movements of the vocal folds, including ejection of air between the folds during closure motion. See p. 15.

189

E2.3 See p. 19.

E2.4 See p. 21.

E2.5 Time-varying glottal impedance affects formants; pitch affects larynx height, so altering length of pharynx; vibration of vocal folds is affected by F_1 resonance.

E2.6 Losses in vocal tract, such as from wall movements, viscosity, heat conduction losses; nasal coupling; loss from radiation to outside air; time-varying loss from glottal impedance. The effects of all these losses depend on what vowel is being produced.

E2.7 The information in a speech signal is mainly conveyed by variation of the frequencies of the main resonances, and of the fundamental frequency. The inherent frequency analysis in spectrograms means that these properties are more clearly seen there than in waveforms.

E2.8 See p. 29 and Figs. 2.10 and 2.11.

E2.9 See pp. 34–36.

E2.10 The main acoustic effects, such as formant frequencies and intensities, depend on many articulatory features, which are difficult to model accurately. The problem is exacerbated by difficulties in measuring human articulation. See p. 32.

CHAPTER 3

E3.1 The peak response from PTCs corresponds with the resonant peak in the basilar membrane, but is much sharper. Neural interactions are believed to be the main cause of the enhanced selectivity — see pp. 44–47.

E3.2 The main effect is probably caused by differences in the amount of phase-locking between the responses of auditory neurons. Some increase of dynamic range could also be given by the fact that hair cells are not all equally sensitive.

E3.3 See section 3.6 (p. 47).

E3.4 See pp. 44, 46–47 and section 3.7.2 (p. 49).

E3.5 Auditory models will make available the information that humans can use, but will discard other information. It is dangerous to use consistent properties of speech production that humans do not use in perception, because they may not be preserved under the influence of what would be judged to be tolerable distortions of a speech signal.

CHAPTER 4

E4.1 See p. 55.

E4.2 Because the quantizing noise is then highly correlated with the speech signal. See p. 56.

E4.3 Auditory masking (see Chapter 3) means that it is more efficient to make quantizing noise vary with signal level.

E4.4 The essential features of a vocoder are: (i) separation of the fine detail from the general shape of the short-term spectrum; (ii) representing the general spectrum shape by a slowly-varying parametric model; (iii) representing periodicity (when present) of excitation by a slowly varying parameter; (iv) re-synthesis from the parametric spectrum model, fed with the signal from an excitation model.

E4.5 The idealizing assumptions of LPC are not well satisfied by real speech (see p. 62). Auditory analysis (see Chapter 3), which is in some ways like channel vocoder analysis with a very large number of channels, appears to be able to cope quite well with the channel approximations to a speech spectrum (see Fig. 4.4).

E4.6 Transmission rate can be reduced by exploiting redundancy in the basic parametric representation. Correlation between parameters at any time can be exploited by vector quantization, and correlation over time can be exploited by variable-frame-rate transmission. The latter inherently needs buffer delay for constant-rate real-time links.

E4.7 See section 4.4.3 (p. 66).

CHAPTER 5

E5.1 Advantages: easy to achieve high technical quality of waveform reproduction; low cost equipment, except for memory costs. Disadvantages: large memory requirement, prosody problems and co-articulation prevent flexibility of message structure.

E5.2 Saving in memory for message storage; ability to modify prosody of stored speech; crude model of co-articulation possible.

E5.3 Advantages: unlimited vocabulary possible with modest memory requirement; straightforward process to change speaker-type or language; provides some aspects of natural articulatory transitions. Disadvantages: limited by quality of vocoder method employed; difficulties of matching diphones at joins; editing new diphones is labour-intensive.

CHAPTER 6

E6.1 See pp. 82–83.

E6.2 Cost of memory for tables is insignificant; initial values for table entries can be guided by phonetic theory, and particularly values can then be changed where shown to be necessary; transformations can be applied to whole sets of tables to change speaker type.

E6.3 Intrinsic allophonic variation is best provided by having co-articulatory effects built into the rule structure; extrinsic allophones can be selected according to the identities of neighbouring phonemes.

E6.4 See p. 86.

E6.5 The fundamental frequency pattern is most important for naturalness, although human productions show quite wide variations. Durations affect phonemic cues as well as stress and rhythm. Intensity variations, except those intrinsic to phoneme type, are of much less importance. See also p. 6.

E6.6 Dictionary look-up is necessary for a high proportion of words, supplemented by spelling-to-sound rules for the inevitable words that will not be covered by the dictionary. See pp. 95–98 for more detail.

E6.7 Because synthesis from concept can provide much information about the required prosody, which is difficult to derive from conventional text.

E6.8 See p. 99.

CHAPTER 7

E7.1 See p. 102. If a suitable distance metric is used, the right word, even though matching poorly, will usually give a better match than other words.

E7.2 Variation of vocal effort, amplifier gain and distance from the microphone mainly cause a scale factor change to the signal. Logarithmic representation converts this to a constant addition to all channels, that does not change the shape of the spectral cross section. Difficulties arise in silences and stop consonent gaps, where the logarithmic level will vary extensively with background noise level.

E7.3 Appropriate orthogonal transformations can reduce the correlation between spectral features and concentrate the important variation in a smaller number of features, so reducing the necessary computation in pattern matching. The main disadvantage is that they prevent the use of subsequent non-linear processing to allow for varying background noise.

E7.4 See pp. 111–113 and Fig. 7.3.

E7.5 Normalization for path length and template length are required. See pp. 113–114.

E7.6 The effects of end-point errors can be mitigated by allowing more freedom for time scale distortion at template ends, and by discounting mismatch at the template end frames. Use of a connected-word algorithm in conjunction with a silence template avoids the problem (see p. 121).

E7.7 See p. 120 and top of p. 121.

E7.8 By tracing back through the optimum path to see where it moves between templates.

E7.9 See p. 122–123.

E7.10 The use of wild-card templates in a training syntax is an effective method (p. 124). For connected-word recognition the performance is much improved by careful choice of syntaxes for embedded training, in which existing word templates precede and follow the wild-card.

CHAPTER 8

E8.1 The features emitted do not uniquely determine the state of the model, which is therefore hidden from the observer.

E8.2 The use of a recurrence relationship enables the state probabilities to be determined successively, from frame to frame.

E8.3 The Viterbi algorithm only considers the likelihood of the most likely path through the model, which must be less than the sum of likelihoods over all possible paths. The practical advantages are in simplifying computation, avoiding scaling problems and simplifying word sequence determination for connected words.

E8.4 The model topology can be constrained by setting some initial transition probabilities to zero. Unsuitable initial values of other parameters may cause a very poor local optimum to be obtained.

E8.5 The main use is to reduce the number of different feature vectors, so that sensible statistical distributions can be obtained from acceptable amounts of training data.

E8.6 See pp. 143–145.

E8.7 When successive states have similar output probability distributions, alternative paths through the states will have similar likelihoods of producing the observed data. The true likelihood can then be many times the maximum (i.e. Viterbi) likelihood. However, this difference between the algorithms will only be obtained if the models are well trained. With a generous allocation of states a very large number of training examples would normally be needed to achieve significant benefit.

E8.8 See top of p. 149.

E8.9 See pp. 149–150.

E8.10 If insufficient training data is available, *a priori* knowledge of variability can be more reliable than measurements from the available data. In particular, the training data for some features may by chance show much less variability than would normally occur.

CHAPTER 9

E9.1 See pp. 155–156.

E9.2 See pp. 156–157.

E9.3 See pp. 159–160.

E9.4 Knowledge of valid words in the language is essential for interpreting phonemic strings into words in connected-word recognition because word boundaries would otherwise be unknown. In realistic recognizers many phonemes will be uncertain or erroneous, so making a dictionary essential even for isolated words. With a dictionary, it is possible to choose the word that fits best in each position by taking into account both acoustic and linguistic evidence.

E9.5 See pp. 161–162.

E9.6 See pp. 162–163.

E9.7 See p. 166. The use of synthesis by rule for recognition essentially involves matching synthetic models of possible utterances against the incoming speech, using a suitable distance metric. The rule system would not have to generate an actual speech signal, but instead could produce a parametric representation appropriate for the distance metric employed. The main potential benefits are removal of irrelevant variation and provision of a model of co-articulation between words.

CHAPTER 10

E10.1 Much of the information needed to produce the appropriate style of speech for synthesis can only be derived from the meaning of the required message. Similarly, the meaning is frequently essential to resolve the choice between alternative utterances in recognition, that are not significantly distinct from the other available evidence. This requirement for understanding is not caused merely by a deficiency in the technology: understanding is intrinsically necessary, and has to be used also by human beings doing the same speech production and recognition tasks.

E10.2 See p. 178.

INDEX